Mayada JEMAA
Sabrine TOUAITI

Herbal Medicine in Endodontic Practice

Mayada JEMAA
Sabrine TOUATI

Herbal Medicine in Endodontic Practice

ScienciaScripts

Imprint

Any brand names and product names mentioned in this book are subject to trademark, brand or patent protection and are trademarks or registered trademarks of their respective holders. The use of brand names, product names, common names, trade names, product descriptions etc. even without a particular marking in this work is in no way to be construed to mean that such names may be regarded as unrestricted in respect of trademark and brand protection legislation and could thus be used by anyone.

Cover image: www.ingimage.com

This book is a translation from the original published under ISBN 978-620-6-71299-2.

Publisher:
Sciencia Scripts
is a trademark of
Dodo Books Indian Ocean Ltd. and OmniScriptum S.R.L publishing group

120 High Road, East Finchley, London, N2 9ED, United Kingdom
Str. Armeneasca 28/1, office 1, Chisinau MD-2012, Republic of Moldova, Europe
Printed at: see last page
ISBN: 978-620-8-26626-4

CONTENTS

INTRODUCTION

Phytotherapy is the study of the use of extracts of natural origin as medicines or agents beneficial to health. [70] For many years, plant-based products have been used in medical and dental practices, and have become even more popular today because of their high antimicrobial activity, biocompatibility and effects. lesser secondary effects. [8] Herbs have interesting medical and physicochemical properties due to the presence of various active principles such as alkaloids, volatile essential oils, glycosides, resins, oleoresins, steroids, tannins, terpenes and phenols. [99] Phytotherapy has been used in the treatment of oral and dental diseases for its anti-inflammatory, antibacterial, antifungal, analgesic and anxiolytic properties, and has been exploited particularly in endodontics to develop safe, effective and economical alternative medical products. [133] The aim of root canal treatment is to achieve maximum disinfection of the root canals. Bacterial reduction is achieved partly by shaping the canals, but mainly by irrigation and intra-canal medication. Complete sterilisation of the endodontium is not easy due to the extremely complex anatomy and the persistence of resistant bacteria in the dentinal tubules. In fact, facultative micro-organisms such as Enterococcus Faecalis, aerobes such as Staphylococcus Aureus and yeasts such as Candida Albicans are considered to be the most resistant species. and the possible causes of failure of endodontic treatment in certain clinical situations. [66] Some conventional endodontic products may present undesirable effects such as tissue toxicity, allergic potential and microbial resistance. [33] Consequently, researchers are increasingly interested in phytopharmaceutical products with different potential applications in endodontics. Indeed, plant-based alternatives could be used as pulp capping or pulpotomy materials, root canal irrigants, intracanal medications, conservation media for permanent teeth avulsed following trauma and also as sealing materials during root canal obturation or in endodontic retreatment. In addition, research evaluating the use of phytotherapy in bone and endodontic regeneration is promising. The aim of our work is to explore the use of phytotherapy in endodontics, focusing on three main areas:

- Definition and historical context of phytotherapy.

- Clinical applications of phytotherapy in endodontics.

- Undesirable effects and drug interactions.

GENERAL NOTIONS ON PHYTOTHERAPY

1. Definition

Phytotherapy, from the Greek phyton, "plant" and therapeia, "treatment", is a treatment modality using plants or products containing them.

According to the World Health Organisation (WHO), phytotherapy is defined as a material or preparation derived from plants which contains raw or processed ingredients of one or more plants with therapeutic values.

Plant-based preparations are derived from a variety of sources, including roots, seeds, leaves, stems and flowers.

Today, we use the term "phytotherapy" to refer to treatment using plants. However, there seems to be a distinction between two concepts:

- **Modern phytotherapy**: based on scientific and biochemical knowledge, its main aim is to relieve symptoms using active ingredients identified in medicinal plants and clinically tested. The products used are often plant extracts presented in the form of pharmaceutical specialities.

- **Traditional" phytotherapy**: this is based on empirical and ancestral practices, using the effects of the whole plant to act on the body as a whole. [78]

2. History

The history of phytotherapy goes back to the origins of mankind. For a long time, people have been harvesting plants not only for food, but also to relieve their ailments.

❖ **The 1st traces of the use of medicinal plants :**

The oldest document to testify to the use of plants in medicine is the Sumerian pharmacopoeia of Nippur, dated 2200 BC. It is a collection of medicinal plants and remedies from the animal and mineral world, engraved on a clay tablet written by the Sumerians in cuneiform characters. [42]

Further evidence of the ancient use of medicinal plants comes from Egypt. The Ebers Papyrus, written in Thebes in 1600 BC, is the first known collection devoted to medicinal plants. At 110 pages, it is by far the most voluminous in ancient Egypt, citing more than 700 names of drugs, including sedatives such as opium, Indian hemp and mandrake, and purgatives such as senna and castor-oil. [42]

India is the world's largest producer of medicinal herbs, known as the "Botanical Garden of the World" [70].

In India, around 20,000 species of medicinal plants have been recorded. However, more than 500 traditional communities use around 800 plant species to treat various illnesses. In this respect, India occupies a unique position in the world, where a number of recognised indigenous systems of medicine, namely Ayurveda, Siddha, Unani, Homeopathy, Yoga and

Naturopathy. [70]Ayurveda, or "Ayurvedic Medicine", is considered to be the oldest holistic medicine in the world. It considers the whole person (body and mind). The Ayurvedic tradition is thought to date back over 5,000 years.

There are about 1250 Indian medicinal plants that are used in the formulation of beneficial measures depending on the Ayurvedic or other ethnic group. [70]

❖ **Plants in Antiquity :**

It was in Greece, around 400 BC, that Western medicine was really born under the impetus of Hippocrates. [42] We attribute to him the writing of all the documents in the Corpus Hippocraticum, and even if it seems that Hippocrates was not the author of all these documents (in view of the disparity of their content), it is nevertheless an important testimony to the practices and knowledge of the art of healing at that time. [78]

This work also introduced the theory of the four humours (the theory that health depends on the balance between the four humours present in the body: blood, bile, pituitary and atrabile) and the notion of Naturamedicatrix, which can be summed up in the fact that the resources for healing are to be found in nature, and the doctor is only there to help the body re-establish its natural balance.

Remedies are used according to the therapeutics of opposites, always with the aim of restoring this balance (for example, cholagogues are used to eliminate an excess of bile). [78]

Over the following centuries, the Greek Empire saw the development of science in many fields, including medicine and botany. Aristotle, the famous scientist and philosopher, was interested in anatomy and physiology. His disciple, Theophrastus, is considered to be the greatest botanist of Antiquity. His works, such as "Historia Plantarum" and "De Causis Plantarum", led to a better understanding of the medicinal properties of plants and enabled them to be classified according to their characteristics[78].

The Romans also used many plants. References to them can be found in Dioscorides' De Materia Medica, a catalogue of medicinal plants. This treatise, which lists all the known drugs of the ancient world, earned its author the reputation of being the father of pharmacognosy.[1] [42]

The second great medical figure was GALIAN (end of the second century), whose influences were largely Hippocratic, since he took up the theory of the four humours and made it more complex, as well as the notion of therapeutics using opposites.

In the second century, he wrote the work "La composition des médicaments", which described and manufactured more than 400 plant-based medicines. It is to him that we owe the term "Galenics", the part of pharmacy that deals with the shaping of pharmaceutical products. [78]

❖ **The Middle Ages :**

The Middle Ages marked the golden age of Arab herbalism. In the course of their many invasions, the Arabs added to their own knowledge the therapeutic heritage of Greek, Latin, Assyrian, Hebrew and Persian civilisations. Ibn Sina, known in Latin as Avicenna, was the greatest physician and philosopher of his time in the 11th century. His encyclopaedic work on medieval medicine, the Kitâb al-Qânoun fi al-Tibb (Canon of Medicine), describes, among other things, the properties and uses of more than 800 medicinal plants. [78]

Technological innovations have led to improvements in distillation techniques and the emergence of new pharmaceutical forms, for example, the discovery of cane sugar, which is used to make syrups. The individualisation of the pharmaceutical profession began with the emergence of the Sayadila. In fact, this profession had originated in Baghdad and was subject to strict rules defined in the Grabadins (in the Arab world, this word refers to a set of texts governing pharmaceutical preparations, the modern equivalent of which is the pharmacopoeia). In Europe, every place of worship had a botanical garden in which the main medicinal plants, known at the time as "simples", were grown. Some figures stand out for their literary contributions, such as Hildegarde of Bingen (1098-1179), author of several works on the properties of medicinal plants. In the rest of the world, the first schools of medicine were founded, and the great civilisations developed their own herbal medicine traditions (Chinese, Mayan, Inca, Aztec, etc.).

It was also during this period that trade developed between Europe, the Middle East, India and Asia, which amplified discoveries and facilitated the exchange of plants between countries [42]

❖ The Renaissance: the golden age of plants

The great expeditions of the late fifteenth century, in particular the discovery of the Americas and the sea route to India, led to new advances as exotic drugs and spices from distant continents converged in Europe. [42] The Spanish introduced cinchona, lemon verbena, tobacco, sarsaparilla and many other plants for food and medicinal use to the old continent.

A century later, Paracelsus revolutionised the small world of herbalists. This Swiss alchemist, astrologer and physician, to whom we owe the famous formula
"Everything is poison, nothing is poison, it is the dose that makes the poison", was considered a precursor of Modern Toxicology. [87]

He was the first to define the foundations of the "Signature Theory": according to this theory, the resemblance between the colour, morphology and biology of many plants and parts of the human body is not due to chance. [87]

❖ Pharmacopoeia of Modern Times :

In Europe, plants were the mainstay of the pharmacopoeia until the end of the 19th century and the advent of modern chemistry. Knowledge of the active components of plants and their therapeutic properties was increasing rapidly, and many active principles of plant origin had been isolated: morphine was isolated from the opium poppy by Friedrich Wilhelm Sertürner (a German pharmacist) in 1804, quinine from cinchona bark in 1820, and alkaloids (nitrogen-based molecules of mainly plant origin) from rye ergot in 1875. [42] In 1838, salicylic acid the chemical precursor of aspirin (acetylsalicylic acid), was extracted from white willow. It was first synthesised in the laboratory in 1860. Since then, phytotherapy and synthetic medicines have followed different paths. Aspirin was created in Germany in 1899 from meadowsweet. For the first time, chemistry improved a natural compound to increase its effectiveness. [87]

In the second half of the 19th century, this process developed and pharmaceutical chemistry was born. [42]For thousands of years, phytotherapy has been the main source of remedies for many illnesses.

In the 19th century, with the discovery of new medicines considered to be miraculous (such as antibiotics), phytotherapy was relegated to the background as "grandmother's remedies" with uncertain virtues. But this sidelining only lasted for a while. The harmful side-effects of some synthetic drugs and resistance to antibiotic therapy soon became apparent. As a result, new research began to focus on plants. [87]

CLINICAL APPLICATIONS OF PHYTOTHERAPY IN ENDODONTICS

1. Preservation of pulp vitality

In vitro and in vivo scientific data have shown promising results for the use of plant extracts in pulp capping or pulpotomy procedures. However, clinical data are rather limited.

❖ Propolis :

Propolis is a natural substance with a resinous consistency resembling wax harvested by Apis Mellifera worker bees from the buds and bark of certain trees **(Figure 1).**

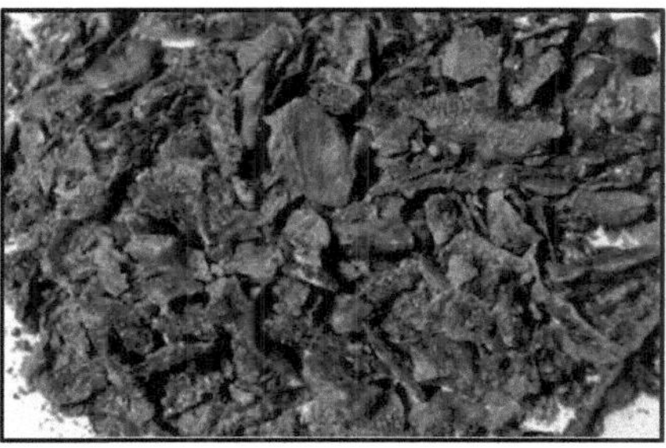

Figure 1: Propolis pieces [186].

Bees use it to strengthen and protect their hives against micro-organisms, repair their structure and cover bee nests. It has been widely used in folk medicine for centuries.

The ancient Greeks, Romans and Egyptians knew about the curative properties of propolis and used it extensively as a medicine.

Its chemical composition varies according to the country of origin, the botanical source and the time of harvest. It is generally made up of : 40 to 55% resins, 20 to 35% beeswax and fatty acids, 10% aromatic oils, 5% pollen, and other components such as minerals and vitamins, its main constituents are flavonoids. [157] Flavonoids are natural molecules belonging to the polyphenol family. They are found in various parts of the plant, in fruit, flowers and leaves and are characterised by their antioxidant, anti-inflammatory, anti-cancer and anti-viral activity. [70]

Due to the complex structure of propolis, it cannot be used directly and must be extracted using an appropriate solvent. Ethanol is the most widely used in published studies because it can produce a propolis extract that is low in wax and rich in biologically active compounds [12]

Propolis is known to be an antioxidant, antimicrobial, anti-inflammatory and cariostatic agent as well as being an excellent immunostimulant. It also has an effect on tissue regeneration and wound healing. [157] According to a study by Bretz et al in 1998, the results showed that there was no significant difference in direct pulp capping with propolis compared to calcium hydroxide products in rats. Both offered a similar degree of inflammation, reducing the amount of microbes and stimulating the creation of a dentinal bridge. [152]

Similarly, it was shown by Sabir et al in 2005 that rat dental pulp capped with propolis had a delayed inflammatory response compared with zinc oxide capsules and stimulated dentin repair compared with control material. [121]

Parolia et al in 2010 conducted a comparative histological analysis of the human pulp following direct pulp capping of 36 premolars with 3 different materials: **Dycal®** (calcium hydroxide paste), **propolis** and **Mineral Trioxide Aggregate (MTA)**. [109]
The aim of this analysis was to study the response of human pulp tissue mechanically exposed to a new material, 'propolis', and to compare it with two existing and commonly used pulp capping agents (**MTA** and **Dycal®**).

The differences in inflammatory response and dentine bridge formation of the pulp exposed to the three different materials were calculated statistically using the chi-square test and were found to be non-significant. Histologically, there was more pulp inflammation in teeth treated with **Dycal®** than with Propolis and MTA on days 15 and 45. In addition, propolis showed results comparable to those obtained with MTA and **Dycal®** in terms of dentine bridge formation. **(Figures 2, 3, 4, 5, 6 and 7).**

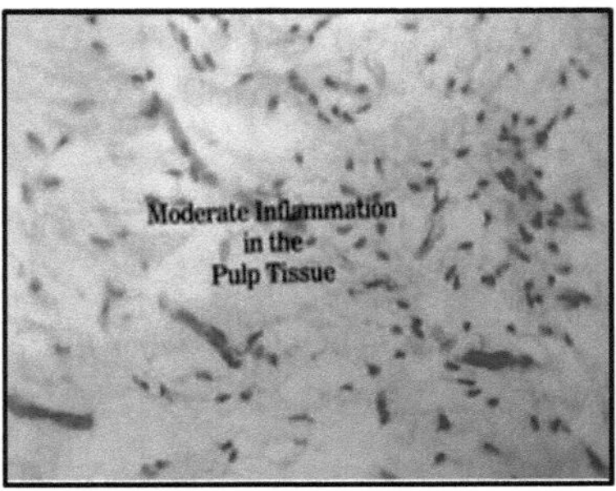

Figure 2: Pulp capping with DYCAL®. No dentine bridge formation and moderate inflammation after 15 days. [109]

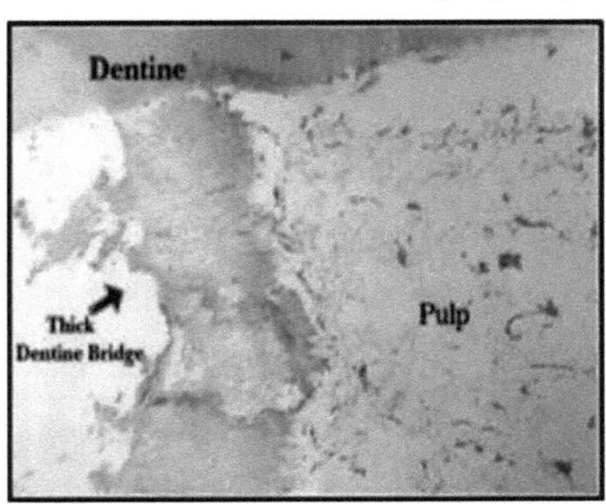

Figure 3: Pulp capping with DYCAL®. Formation of a thick dentine bridge after 45 days. (The arrow indicates the dentine bridge) [109].

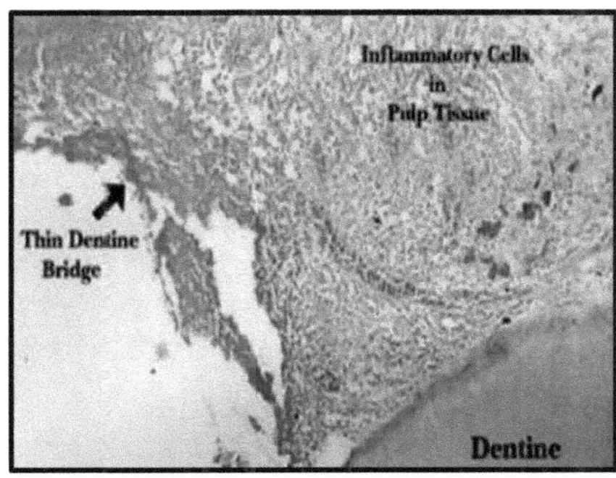

Figure 4: Propolis pulp capping. Formation of a thin dentine bridge after 15 days. (The arrow indicates the dentine bridge) [109].

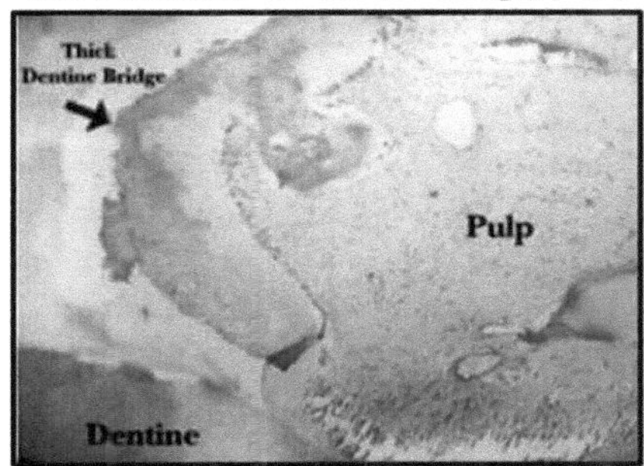

Figure 5: Propolis pulp capping. Formation of a thick dentine bridge after 45 days. (The arrow indicates the dentine bridge) [109].

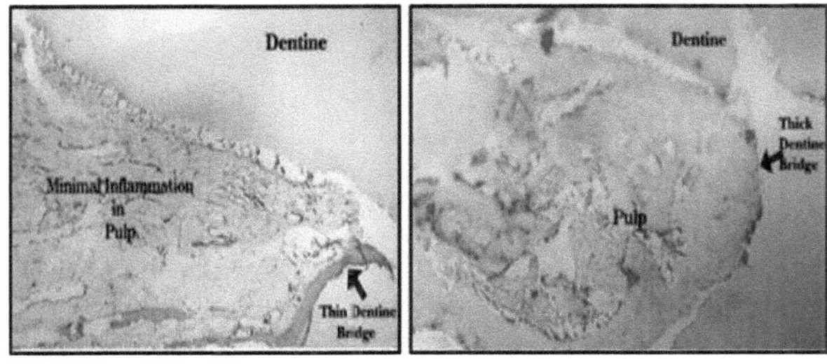

Figure 6: Pulpal plug with MTA, formation of a thin calcified bridge after 15 days. [109]

Figure 7: Pulpal plug with MTA. Formation of a thick dentine bridge after 45 days. [109]

Propolis thanks to its anti-inflammatory action inhibits prostaglandin synthesis and helps the immune system by promoting phagocytic activity and stimulating cellular immunity (Balata et al 2018). [33] Stimulation of various enzyme systems, cell metabolism, circulation and collagen formation could contribute to the formation of hard tissue bridges by Propolis. These effects are the result of the presence of arginine, vitamin C, a provitamin A and B complex and trace elements such as copper, iron and zinc, as well as bioflavonoids. [109]
Ahangari et al in 2012, found that dental pulp from guinea pigs capped with propolis induced the production of high quality tubular dentin in 100% of the cases studied while 14% of the calcium hydroxide cases produced porous dentin. Added to this, the propolis group showed no signs of inflammation, infection or necrosis and that propolis stimulated stem cell production. [152]

In 2015, Kusum et al clinically and radiographically evaluated the efficacy of mineral trioxide aggregates **(MTA)**, **Biodentine** and **Propolis** in pulpotomy of deciduous teeth. The results showed that clinical and radiographic success rates over a 9-month period in the 3 groups were 92, 80 and 72%, respectively. [157]

A randomised clinical trial conducted by Ahangari et al in 2021 aimed to evaluate propolis as a pulp capping material compared to calcium hydroxide on human teeth. The results of this study revealed two different types of dentin. Calcium hydroxide induced the formation of low-quality reparative dentin with voids that resembled bone tissue called osteodentin. But, the newly formed dentin induced by propolis was high-quality dentin containing tubules that can act as a barrier against the invasion of microbial pathogens and prevent pulpal damage. [10]

In addition to its anti-inflammatory effect, propolis has been shown to play an important role in reducing dentinal permeability and hypersensitivity. This characteristic results from the fact that bee glue has the ability to partially impregnate dentinal tubules. [152] At present, scientific data is fairly limited as to the superiority of propolis over other therapeutics. in pulp capping. Consequently, clinical studies with a high level of scientific proof seem necessary.

❖ **Nigella (Nigella Sativa) :**

Nigella Sativa, also known as "black seed" or "cumin", is an aromatic plant in the Renonculaceae family **(Figure 8)**. [105]

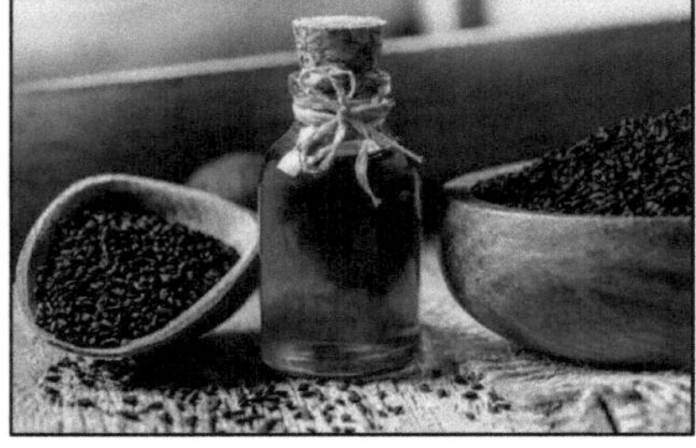

Figure 8. Black cumin seeds [176]

Many medicinal uses of this plant have been scientifically tested, and some have been confirmed. In particular, black seed extract has been shown to possess numerous pharmacological properties. In fact, this extract is a bronchodilator, anti-carcinogen, antioxidant, hypotensive, analgesic, antibacterial and anti-inflammatory. [105] Concerns about the side effects of formocresol as a pulpotomy agent in paediatric dentistry have led to a search for new drugs. Formocresol contains formaldehyde, which is classified as a known mutagenic, cytotoxic and human carcinogenic compound by the World Health Organization (WHO) and the International Agency for Research on Cancer (IARC). In this context, Omar et al in 2012 carried out a histopathological study on dog teeth to assess the pulp reaction to black cumin oil and formocresol. The results of this study showed that NS oil has an anti-inflammatory effect and the pulp retains its vitality after application. This could qualify its use as a pulpotomy medication for primary teeth. [105] However, a study conducted by Sara Hashem et al in 2019 evaluating the use of Nigella Sativa, Miswak and Allium Sativum(Garlic) in pulpotomy procedures of human primary teeth concluded that Allium Sativum and Miswak can be considered as a good natural alternative to formocresol unlike NS which showed absence of dentin bridge in histopathological examination. [65]

▪ Turmeric (Curcuma Longa) :

Turmeric (Curcuma Longa) is a short-stemmed perennial plant with large, oblong leaves and oval, pear-shaped or oblong rhizomes that are often branched and brownish-yellow **in colour (Figure 9)**.A member of the Zingiberaceae family, it is grown in several regions of the Indian subcontinent, South-East Asia and South America.Its active ingredient is curcumin, which acts as a powerful anti-oxidant and anti-inflammatory agent by inhibiting lipoxygenase and cyclooxygenase. [8]

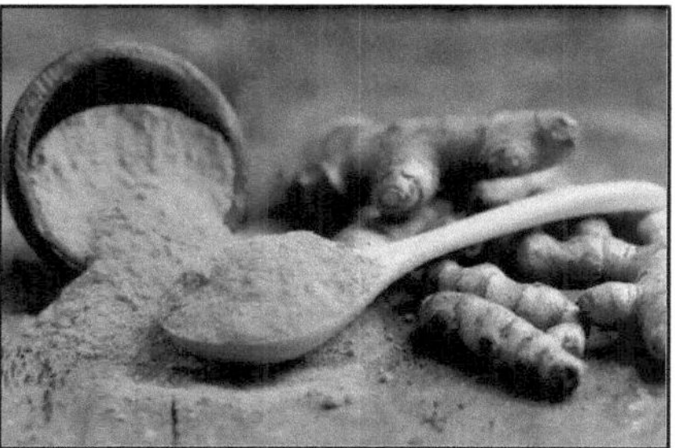

Figure 9: Turmeric powder [174].

Mandrol et al in 2016 conducted a study evaluating the cytotoxicity of curcumin against dental pulp fibroblasts on primary teeth, the authors found that curcumin promotes cell viability and induces proliferation of primary dental pulp fibroblasts and has the potential to be developed into a cost-effective and reliable drug for vital pulp therapy. [88] Due to its medicinal properties, turmeric powder mixed with distilled water was used as a pulpotomy medication in primary teeth by Purohit et al in 2017, on 50 children aged 4 to 9 years with a follow-up of 3 weeks, 2 months, 4 months and 6 months **(Figure 10)**. Pulpotomy with turmeric showed clinical and radiological success, but the authors recommended further studies with histological evaluation. [115]

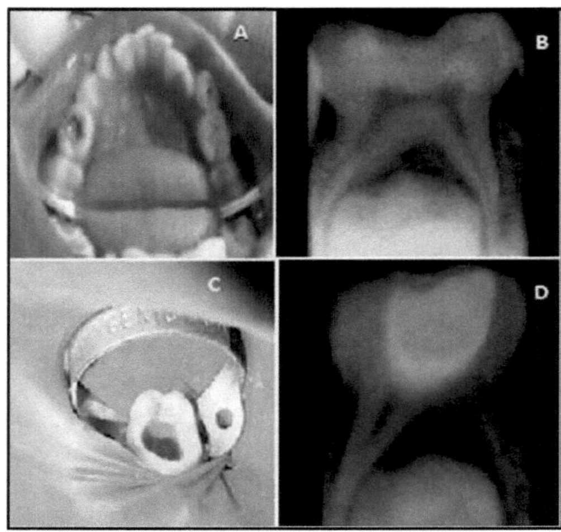

Figure 10: (A): Carious 85;(B): Preoperative radiograph of 85; (C): Turmeric mixed with distilled water placed in 85; (D): Postoperative radiograph after 6 months [115].

Similarly, Hugar et al in 2017 conducted a study to evaluate and compare the clinical pulp response and radiographic signs after pulpotomy in 90 temporary molars treated with formocresol (control), propolis extract, turmeric gel and calcium hydroxide respectively.

After 1 and 3 months, the teeth in all groups were judged to be clinically and radiographically healthy. However, after 6 months, one tooth in experimental group 1 (**Propolis**) showed signs of radiological failure but was clinically asymptomatic.Also, failures in the form of internal resorption were observed on two teeth in experimental group 2 (**turmeric**) **(Figure 11)** which were free of any clinical signs or symptoms.In experimental group 3 (**calcium hydroxide**) four teeth showed radiological failure, 3 of which showed signs of pain **(Figure 12).** All the teeth in the control group (**formocresol**) were judged to be clinically and radiographically healthy after 1, 3 and 6 months. [71]

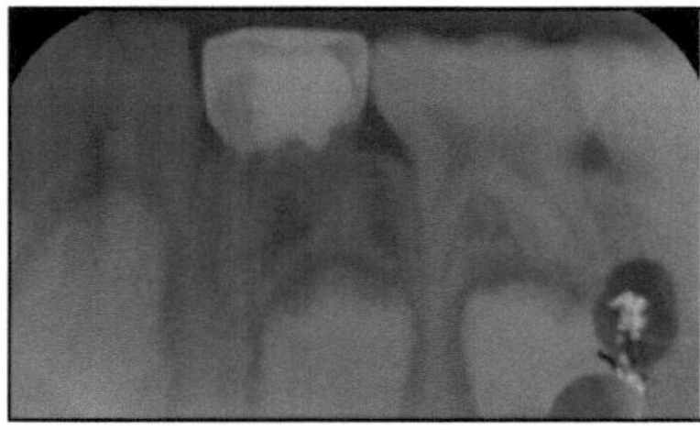

Figure 11: Internal resorption detected in a case treated with turmeric pulpotomy [71].

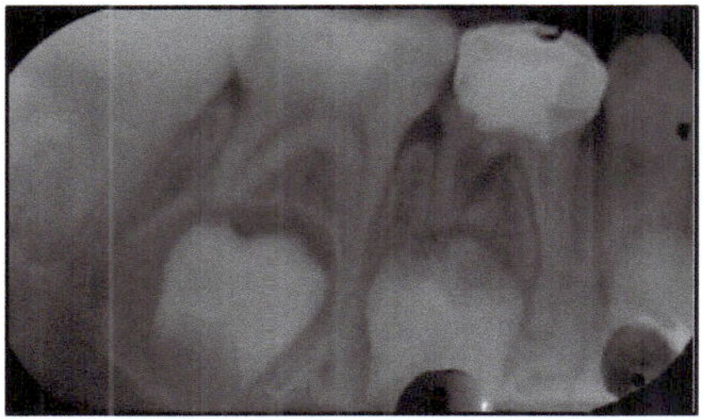

Figure 12: Internal resorption observed in a case treated by pulpotomy with calcium hydroxide [71].

In conclusion, the authors observed acceptable clinical and radiological results with the use of turmeric as a pulpotomy agent in primary molars. However, they recommended a long-term histological analysis to take into account the failures that occurred in the present study. [71]

❖ **Thyme(Thymus Vulgaris) :**

Thymus Vulgaris is a perennial plant native to the Mediterranean region and cultivated in several countries **(Figure 13).** This plant has been used medicinally for thousands of years for its antibacterial, antitussive, spasmolytic and antioxidant properties.

Thymol, one of the ingredients in thyme, is used as an antiseptic in mouthwashes and has been shown to reduce the formation of dental plaque and cavities. [77]

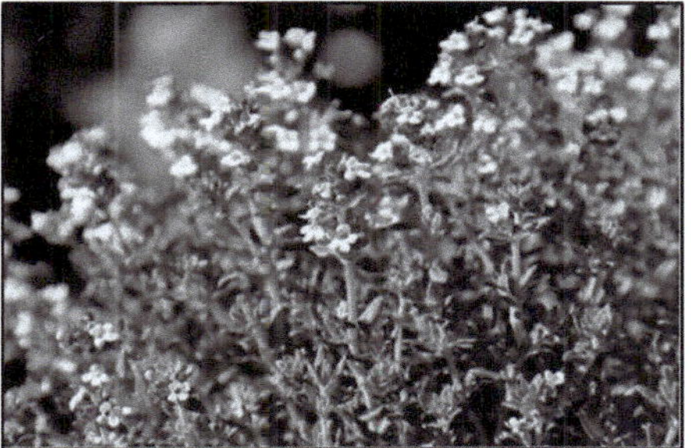

Figure 13: Thyme flowers [159].

Alolofi et al in 2016 performed a clinical and radiographic evaluation of ethanolic extract of thymus vulgaris as a pulpotomy agent in primary molars. The study showed a good clinical success rate of 94.1% at 1, 6 and 12 months. This result was attributed to the antibacterial anti-inflammatory and haemostatic activity of thymus components such as thymol flavonoids, carvacrol and apigenin. [77]

❖ **Garlic (Allium Sativum):**

It is one of the most extensively studied medicinal plants. The antibacterial activity of Allium sativum is due to the Allicin produced by the enzymatic activity of Allinase. It has been reported in the literature that garlic extract inhibits multi-resistant strains of Streptococcus

Mutans isolated from decayed human teeth. [77] Indeed, Mohamed et al in 2015 compared the effects of formocresol and Allium Sativum oil on the pulp tissue of 18 premolars after pulpotomy. The authors found that Allium Sativum oil is a biocompatible material with human pulp tissue. It has good healing potential, leaving the pulp tissue healthy and functional, whereas teeth treated with formocresol showed chronic inflammation leading to necrosis. [98]

❖ **Aloe Vera :**

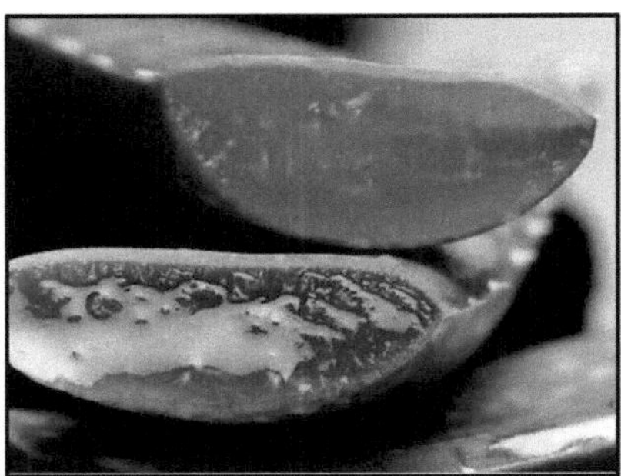

Figure 14: Aloe vera leaves [171].

This herb belongs to the Liliaceae family, also known a s Aloe Barbadensis Mill **(Figure 14).** Aloe has an anti-inflammatory anti-inflammatory, immunomodulating, antibacterial, antifungal and healing action. [77]Its antibacterial activity is due to its ability to inhibit protein synthesis in bacterial cells. [125] Aloe Vera inhibits the cyclooxygenase pathway and reduces the production o f prostaglandin from arachidonic acid. [125] In 2008, Gala-Garcia et al found that applying Aloe vera directly to the pulp tissue of rats resulted in the development of tertiary dentin. This was explained by the presence of various bioactive constituents such as polysaccharides, glycoprotein and beta-sitosterol that stimulate wound healing, angiogenesis and cell proliferation. [77]

Aloe vera was used as a pulpotomy agent by Gupta et al in 2010 on primary molars. The authors found that freshly extracted Aloe Vera gel can be used as an effective pulpotomy agent. [77] In addition, a study by Kalra et al in 2017 evaluated the effect of freshly extracted Aloe vera extract and Mineral Trioxide Aggregate (MTA) as pulpotomy agents in primary molars. Clinical and radiographic evaluation of all pulpotomised teeth was carried out for approximately 12 months, followed by histopathological evaluation. The results showed that pulpotomy with MTA was superior to that with A.Vera plant extract. [77]

However, acemannan, a polysaccharide from Aloe vera, showed similar results to MTA in partial pulpotomy of canine teeth, resulting in the formation of a mineralised bridge with normal pulp tissue without pulp inflammation or necrosis, whereas formocresol showed pulp inflammation without the formation of a mineralised bridge. [138] Acemannan, on the other hand, has been studied as a direct capping material on primary human teeth. This natural product promoted dentin formation by stimulating the proliferation, differentiation, formation and growth of dentin. extracellular matrix formation and mineralisation of primary cells in human dental pulp. [137]

Similarly, according to a study by Tiên Thuy in 2020, acemannan sponges induced continued root formation on immature permanent teeth treated by direct pulp capping or partial pulpotomy. The authors suggested that acemannan is a promising low-cost biomaterial for vital pulp therapy. [150]

2. Irrigation endodontics

The researchers were interested in plant-based products to offset the side-effects of conventional products commonly used in endodontic irrigation. Although sodium hypochlorite (NAOCl) is recommended as an endodontic irrigant for its high antibacterial action and its ability to dissolve necrotic tissue, it is toxic to periapical tissue, corrosive to metals, has allergic potential and an unpleasant taste and odour. In addition, it alters the mechanical properties of dentin by reducing the modulus of elasticity and its flexural strength. [8] Chlorhexidine digluconate (CHX) is used in endodontics at concentrations ranging from 0.12 to 2% because of its broad-spectrum antibacterial properties and substantivity (residual effect). However, it is unable to dissolve organic matter, does not remove dentinal sludge, can cause tooth discolouration and forms a potentially toxic orange-brown precipitate (parachloroaniline) when brought into contact with NaOCl [8]. New irrigants such as BioPure MTAD (a mixture of tetracycline, citric acid and detergent) are an effective solution for removing but has certain disadvantages such as high cost and short shelf life. [48]

❖ Morinda Citrifolia or Noni :

Morinda Citrifolia, commercially known as "Noni" or "Noni". The "Indian mulberry tree", discovered in Polynesia 2000 years ago, is considered an important folk medicine **(Figure 15)**. [21]

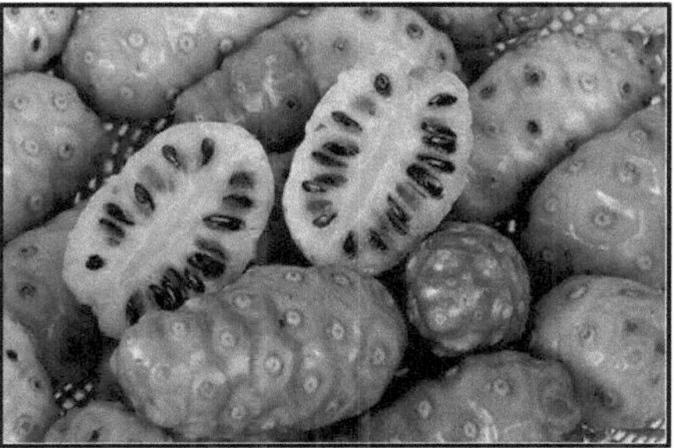

Figure 15: Fruit of Morinda Citrifolia [179].

Indeed, Morinda Citrifolia (MC) has a wide range of therapeutic effects, including antibacterial, antiviral, antifungal, anti-tumour, analgesic, hypotensive, anti-inflammatory and also stimulates the immune system. [102] Morinda citrifolia juice contains antibacterial compounds such as L-asperuloside, Alizarin, Scopoletin, Octanoic acid, Potassium, Vitamin C, terpenoids, alkaloids and anthraquinones. [21] These compounds have been shown to help combat infectious bacterial strains such as Pseudomonas Aeruginosa, Proteus Morgani, Staphylococcus Aureus, Baciillis Subtilis Escherichia coli, Salmonella and Shigella. [21]

Morinda Citrifolia juice acts by depolymerising water-soluble pectins, whereas the pectinases and hemicellulases in the juice of Morinda Citrifolia lead to differential disassembly of bacterial cell wall polymers. [100] Murray et al in 2008 conducted a study to compare the efficacy of Morinda citrifolia juice (MCJ) with sodium hypochlorite (6%) and Chlorhexidine (2%) in t h e removal of dentinal sludge.

The results of this study showed that the "Smear Layer" of root canals was instrumented by scanning electron microscope (SEM) analysis. The minimum inhibitory concentration (MIC) of MCJ on the growth of E. Faecalis in test tubes proved to be a 6% solution. [102]

Murray et al found that 6% Morinda Citrifolia juice was as effective as 6% NAOCL combined with EDTA (17%) in removing dentinal sludge and more effective than 2% CHX.

In fact, CHX was not very effective in removing dentinal sludge and the mixture of CHX and MCJ created one of the least effective irrigation solutions. **(Figure 16)** [102]

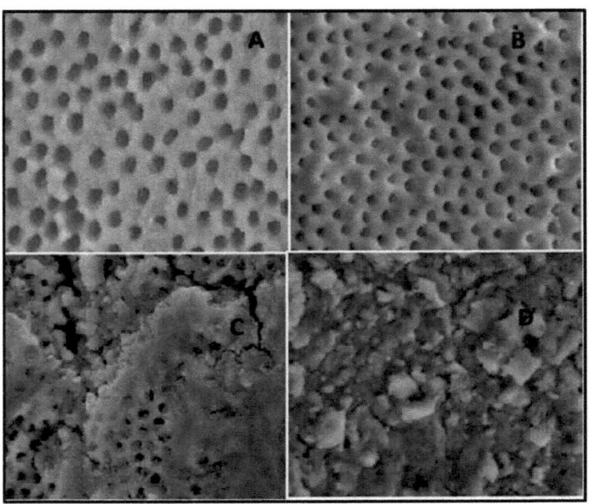

Figure 16: SEM observations of canal walls (magnification *2000) [102].

(A) (A): Irrigation with NaOCL + EDTA, open dentinal tubules;(B): Irrigation with MCJ + EDTA, removal of dentinal sludge, open dentinal tubules. (c): Irrigation with CHX, partial elimination of dentinal sludge, dentinal tubules partially occluded with the presence of a layer of dentinal sludge. (D) Saline irrigation of the root canal, dentin sludge intact.

On the other hand, the authors indicated that CM juice is a biocompatible antioxidant, unlikely to cause serious accidents to patients, unlike NaOCl [102]. Recent studies have reported that long-term exposure (1 hour) to NaOCl may weaken the structural integrity of dentin [8].

While the study by Saghiri et al in 2013 showed that 6% MC juice followed by a final rinse with 17% EDTA is an effective solution for the removal of dentin sludge without any negative influence on the microhardness of root dentin. This is another advantage of MC over NaOCL. [122]

Further studies are needed to assess biocompatibility and safety before Morinda citrifolia extract can be definitively recommended as an intracanal irrigation solution. Indeed, in vitro observations of the efficacy of MC when used with an EDTA flush appear promising. [102]

❖ Propolis :

Because of its anti-inflammatory and anti-bacterial properties, propolis has attracted interest in endodontic research as an irrigant and intracanal medication.The pharmacologically active components of propolis are phenolics, aromatics and flavonoids. [154] Propolis' antibacterial power is due to its high flavonoid content and its anti-inflammatory activity is explained by the presence of caffeic acid and ferulic acid. [154]

It has been reported in the literature that propolis has effective antibacterial and antifungal activity against Actinomyces naeslundi, Fusobaterium nucleatum, Lactosbacillus acidophilus Prevotella oralis, **Porphyromonas** gingivalis, Staphylococcus aureus, Escherichia coli and candida albicans. [33]

The mechanism of propolis' antibacterial activity remains ambiguous. Some authors have stated that it is associated with a synergistic action of its components. [19]

They have suggested that the mechanism of action is based on its inhibitory action on bacterial growth by blocking cell division, by disorganising the cytoplasm, by inhibiting protein synthesis, the adhesion process, the enzymes responsible for bacterial proliferation or by inhibiting nucleic acid synthesis. [19]

In a 2003 comparative study by Al-Qathami and Al-Madi on the antimicrobial efficacy of propolis, 2.5% NaOCl and saline as intracanal irrigants, the authors found that propolis had antimicrobial activity equal to that of 2.5% NaOCl. [19]

Other authors have evaluated the efficacy of propolis on an E.faecalis biofilm model on a dental substrate. The study revealed that propolis had similar antibacterial efficacy to NaOCL (5.25%). [52] Tyagi et al in 2013 studied the antimicrobial efficacy of propolis, Morinda Citrifolia, Azadirachta Indica (Neem) and hypochlorite of sodium hypochlorite (5%) on the Candida Albicans biofilm. The results showed that the sodium hypochlorite (5%) and propolis groups had the greatest antimicrobial efficacy against C. Albicans, followed by the A. Indica (Neem) and M. Citrifolia groups. [145] These results were confirmed by other in vitro studies in which propolis was as effective as NaOCL (5%) and CHX (2%) against Candida albicans and E. faecalis. [26, 24] Although propolis has been shown to be more reliable than NAOCL in terms of biocompatibility, the variation in chemical composition ,extraction methods and methods of assessing antibacterial activity raise concerns about quality control and batch-to-batch variability for the standardised development of new medicines.[94] It would therefore be essential to develop more in vitro and in vivo studies for a more thorough evaluation of propolis as a promising material in endodontic practice. [33]

❖ Azadirachta Indica (Neem) :

Neem is a medicinal tree native to India known as the Neem tree. "Indian Margousier" or 'Indian Lilac". **(Figure 17)** Each part of the tree has been studied in phytotherapy. Medicinal uses have been described, particularly for the leaves, fruit and bark. The leaves contain alkaloids, glycosides, saponins, flavonoids, steroids, anthraquinone and tannic acid, all of which have therapeutic value. Furthermore, it has been described in the literature that Neem has antibacterial, antifungal, antiviral, antioxidant, anti-inflammatory, antipyretic, analgesic and immunostimulant properties. [8,21]

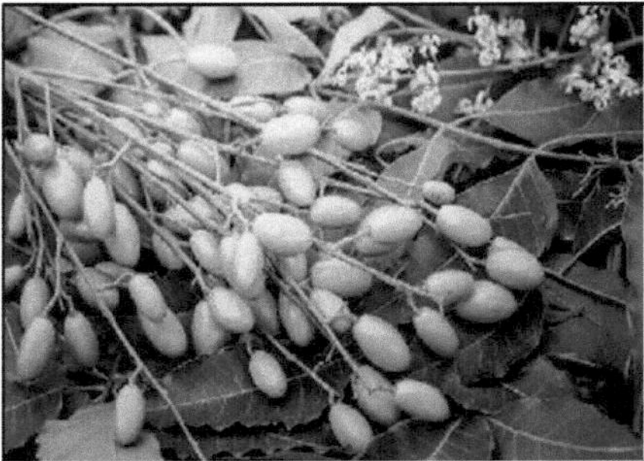

Figure 17: Neem fruits and leaves [167].

Arati et al in 2011 observed that ethanolic extract of Neem had significant antimicrobial activity against E. faecalis. [8]It acts by inhibiting the cell membrane and altering bacterial adhesion to dentine. [100] Compared to a 5.25% sodium hypochlorite solution, Vinothkumar et al in 2013 observed that Neem leaf extract had significant antimicrobial efficacy against Enterococcus faecalis and Candida albicans. [33]Another study by Ghonmode et al in 2013 showed that Neem leaf extract had a significant antimicrobial effect superior to 3 % NaOCL against E.faecalis. [57]

In addition, by comparing the efficacy of various plant extracts, namely green tea extract, orange oil and neem leaf extract, in removing dentinal sludge using electron microscopic analysis at Scanning (SEM), Sebatni et al in 2017 found that the highest efficiency of dentin sludge removal was observed in canals treated with neem leaf extract. [126]

❖ **Triphala :**

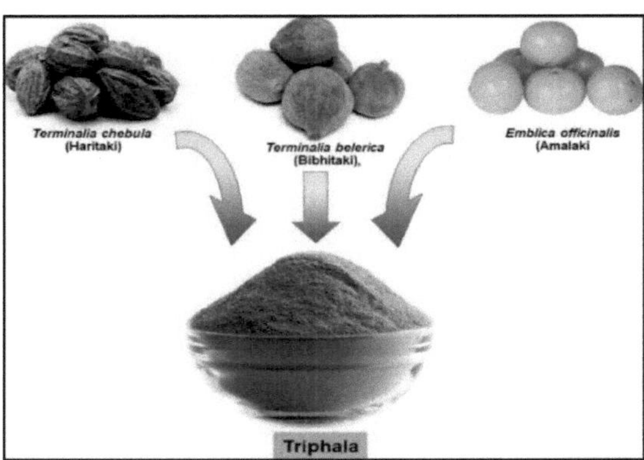

Figure 18: Constituents of Triphala [178].

Triphala is an Ayurvedic herbal formulation comprising dried fruit powders of three medicinal plants Terminalia bellerica, Terminalia chebula and Emblica officinalis **(Figure18)**

Studies have reported that tannic acid, a major constituent of Triphala, has bacteriostatic and bactericidal properties against certain Gram (+) and Gram (-) pathogens. It acts by inactivating microbial adhesins, cell envelope transport proteins and enzymes. [100]

The presence of tannins, quinones, flavoroids, gallic acid and citric acid explains its ability to eliminate the dentine smear layer and its use as a root canal chelator. [143] Added to this, it effectively inhibits biofilm formation thanks to its ability to trap free radicals and its antibacterial power, and is also proving to be an alternative to sodium hypochlorite for endodontic irrigation. [125, 143]

Indeed, according to a comparative study conducted by Divia et al in 2018, Triphala showed antibacterial activity against E. faecalis comparable t o that of 5% NaOCl which is a gold standard for comparison of endodontic irrigants. [45]

Compared to many commonly used root canal irrigants, Triphala has less cytotoxicity. In addition to its antioxidant and anti-inflammatory properties, the fruit juice of Emblica officinalis (a component of Triphala) has the highest vitamin C content and contributes 45-70% to its antioxidant properties. [36]

Although NaOCL has bactericidal properties and is capable of dissolving organic tissues, its ability to remove dentin sludge from the instrumented canal walls has been shown to be insufficient. Thus, Bhargava et al in 2015 conducted a study to compare the efficacy of 3 antioxidants: (Neem, Triphala and Emblica officinalis (Amla) versus NaOCl (5.25%) in combination with EDTA (17%) in removing dentin sludge by SEM analysis. [36] The results of this study showed that Neem, Triphala and Amla had significant potential for eliminating dentine sludge, particularly Amla, which was as effective as NAOCL solution (5.25% combined with EDTA (17%) **(Figure 19, 20, 21, 22,23).**Nevertheless, further investigations are needed to confirm its efficacy as an endodontic irrigant. [36]

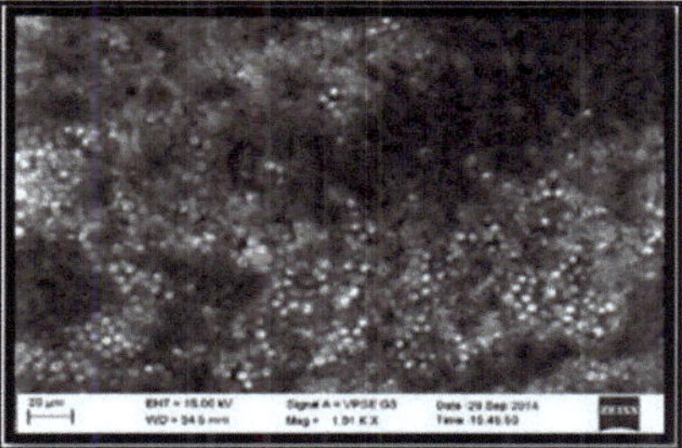

Figure 19: SEM view; Removal of dentin sludge after irrigation with Neem (magnification x 1000) [36].

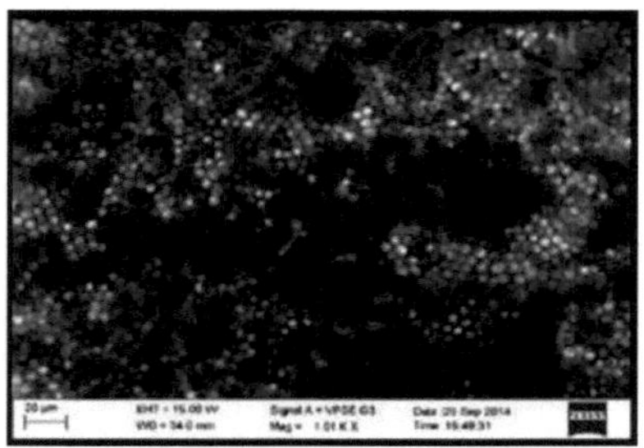

Figure 20: SEM view; Removal of dentinal sludge after irrigation with Triphala. (Magnification x 1000) [36]

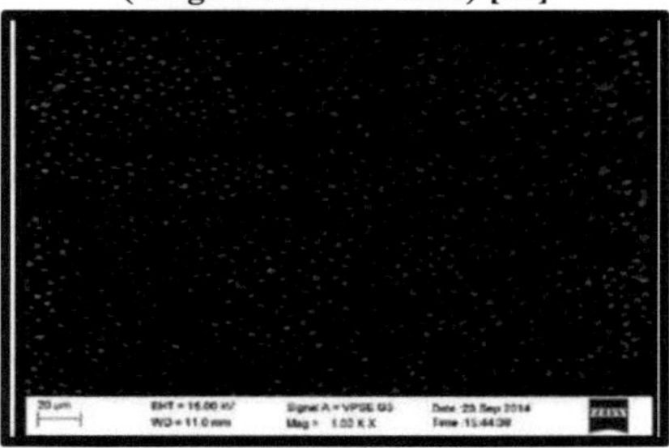

Figure 21: SEM view; Removal of dentin sludge after irrigation with Amla. (Magnification x 1000) [36]

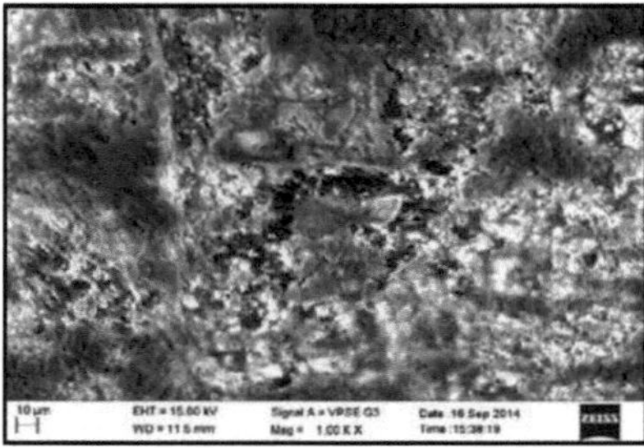

Figure 22: SEM view; Removal of dentin sludge after irrigation with saline solution (magnification x 1000) [36].

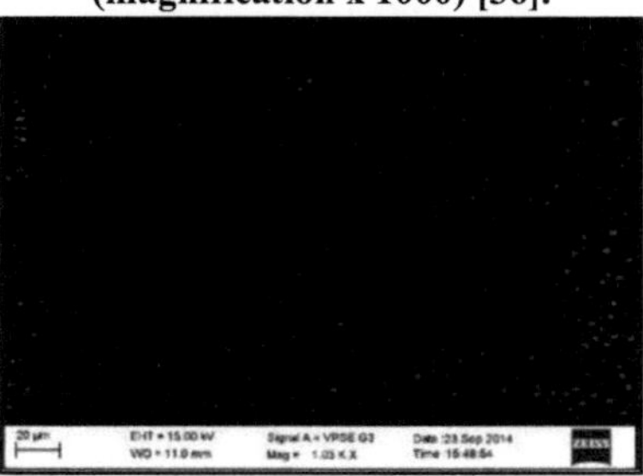

Figure 23: SEM view; Removal of dentin sludge after irrigation with 17% EDTA (magnification x 1000) [36].

- **Green tea (Camellia Sinensis) :**

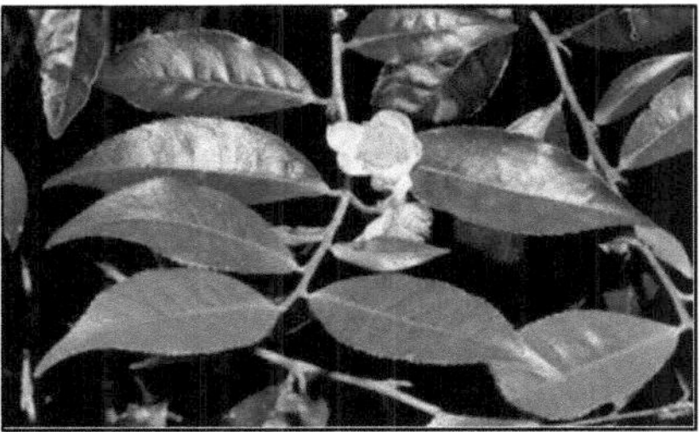

Figure 24: Leaves of Camellia Sinensis [178].

Green tea, extracted from Camellia Sinensis, is widely consumed around the world **(Figure 24)**. Epigallocatechin-3-gallate (EGCG) is the most abundant polyphenol in green tea. Studies have shown that EGCG irreversibly disrupts the membrane of Gram (+) and Gram (-) bacteria and inhibits bacterial DNA gyrase, preventing DNA supercoiling and leading to bacterial cell death.EGCG neutralises toxic terminal metabolites such as collagenase, protein tyrosine phosphatase and alkaline phosphatase from pathogenic bacteria. [52] The interesting properties of green tea such as availability, cost effectiveness, long shelf life, low toxicity and lack of microbial resistance have sparked the interest of researchers to study its effect as an endodontic irrigant. [43]Prabhakar et al in 2010 conducted a study on the antimicrobial efficacy of plant-based alternatives (Triphala and Green Tea Polyphenols (GTP), (MTAD) and NaOCl (5%) against E. faecalis biofilm. It was observed that 5% NaOCL was the most effective antibacterial agent while triphala and green tea had significant antimicrobial activity against E. Faecalis biofilm formed in the dental substrate. [113]

The results of this study are consistent with other studies. According to Garg et al in 2014, propolis and triphala were as effective as NaOCl (5.25%) against E. faecalis biofilm. However, green tea polyphenols showed less efficacy. [52] Similarly, in another in vitro study by Dadresanfar et al in 2019 exploring the antibacterial role of green tea as an endodontic irrigant compared with NaOCl (5.25%) and CHX (2%) in E.faecalis infected root canals, the results of this study showed that the reduction in the number of microorganisms was 100% with NaOCl, 98.9% with CHX, 81% with 12.5% green tea and 94.8% with 25% green tea. [43]To explore the antifungal efficacy of green tea as an endodontic irrigant against C. albicans biofilm, 45 extracted premolars were sectioned vertically and randomly divided into three groups after biomechanical preparation of the root canals. All samples were infected with C. albicans and exposed to the test solutions (sodium hypochlorite (5%), green tea (1%), normal saline) for 5, 10 and 15 minutes. The mean number of C. albicans in the green tea and sodium hypochlorite groups decreased to 25% and 50% of the initial values respectively. Furthermore, according to the present study, the antifungal activity of green tea increased over time. [50] Because of the naturalness of green tea extract, its low toxicity, its reasonable price and the absence o f side effects, the authors have concluded that it could be used as an endodontic irrigation solution. However, further in vivo studies seem necessary.

❖ **Acacia Nilotica Linn (Babool):**

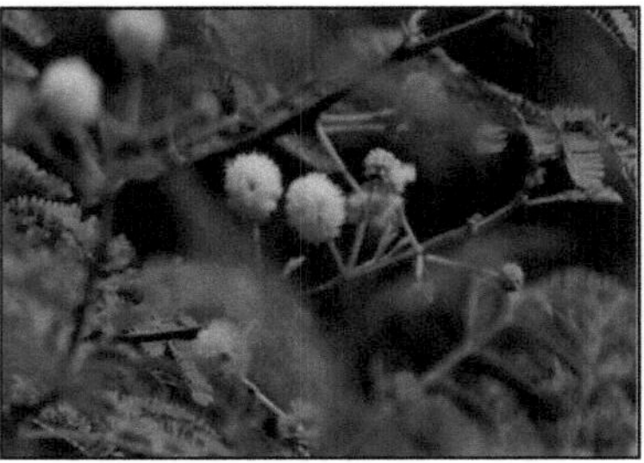

Figure 25: Acacia Nilotica [169]

It is a medicinal plant native to Egypt **(Figure 25).**

It has antimicrobial, antifungal, antiviral, antibiotic, anticancer and antiplatelet properties. It contains anti-inflammatory agents that inhibit the synthesis of prostaglandin, one of the most important mediators of inflammation.Acacia Nilotica extract acts on bacteria by damaging essential electrolytic and cellular constituents (proteins and nucleic acids). [100]In 2019, Payal A Jain et al carried out an in vitro study which aimed to evaluate and compare the antibacterial activity of aqueous extracts of Punica Granatum (Pomegranate bark), Acacia Nilotica (Babool stem bark) and Emblica Officinalis (Amla fruit) against E faecalis and their abilities to remove dentin sludge (Smear layer). [74]Minimum inhibitory concentrations (MICs) of Punica Granatum, Acacia Nilotica and Emblica Officinalis were identified using the broth microdilution method at 6.25%, 25% and 12.5% respectively. An agar well diffusion test was performed and the zones of inhibition were measured to assess antibacterial activity. The highest zone of inhibition was recorded for 6.25% Punica granatum (21 mm), followed by 12.5% Emblica officinalis (20 mm) and the lowest for 25% Acacia nilotica with a zone of inhibition measuring (14 mm) **(Figure26).**

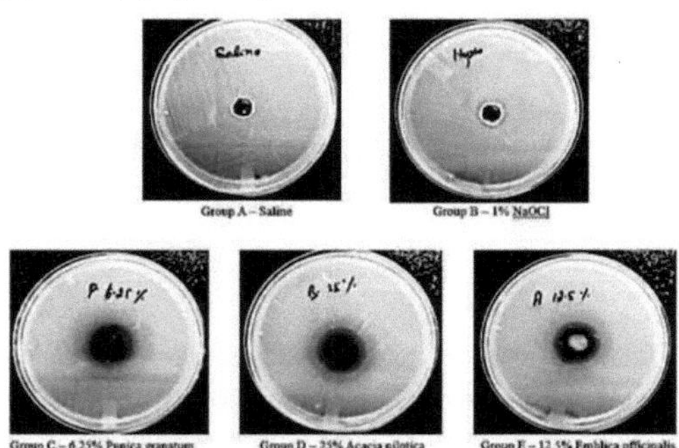

Figure 26: Agar diffusion test showing zones of inhibition in millimetres (mm). [74]

With regard to smear layer removal, scanning electron microscopy (SEM) analysis revealed that Acacia Nilotica had no smear removal properties and its mean scores were similar to those of the negative control groups (0.9% saline solution and 1% sodium hypochlorite solution) while the 6.25% Punica Granatum solution and 12.5% Emblica Officinalis solution were as effective as 17% EDTA in removing dentine sludge. [74] According to a study carried out by Gupta et al in 2020, comparing the antibacterial efficacy of Thymus Vulgaris at 20%, Salvadora Persica at 12.5%, Acacia Nilotica at 10%, Calendula Arvensis at 10% and sodium hypochlorite at 5% in eliminating Enterococcus faecalis, NaOCl (5%) showed the highest antibacterial activity against E. faecalis. The other products also showed significant antibacterial efficacy. These natural products have therefore been proposed as alternatives to 5% NaOCl. [62]

❖ Garlic (Allium Sativum) :

Some studies have suggested that garlic could be an effective alternative to sodium hypochlorite. This is linked to its antibacterial properties. The allicin present in garlic largely destroys the walls and cell membranes of root canal bacteria. (1mg of allicin is equivalent to 15 IU of penicillins). [143,108] A study published by Gopalakrishnan et al in 2014 showed complete inhibition of E. faecalis between the NaOCL 5.25% and CHX 2% groups, while garlic and cinnamon extract showed weaker inhibition compared to these two groups (NaOCL 5.25% and CHX 2%). [33]

These results are consistent with those of an in vitro study which evaluated the antimicrobial efficacy of cinnamon, garlic and turmeric as endodontic irrigants against Enterococcus faecalis and Candida albicans in comparison with 5.25% NaOCL. Garlic showed the highest antibacterial activity, followed by cinnamon and turmeric. Nevertheless, NaOCL showed complete inhibition of E faecalis and Candida albicans, and the authors concluded that it remains the reference irrigant. [108]

In 2015, Birring et al observed that concentrations of garlic extract (10%, 40% and 70%) showed considerable antimicrobial efficacy against E.faecalis. Indeed, the 70% concentration was the most effective and showed similar antimicrobial efficacy to 5.25% NaOCL. [33]

In addition, in a randomised clinical trial conducted by Siddique et al in 2020 to evaluate the antimicrobial action of 1.8% garlic-lemon and 3% sodium hypochlorite (NaOCl) on 30 patients diagnosed with asymptomatic apical periodontitis, garlic-lemon was as effective as sodium hypochlorite in reducing the microbial load. The authors suggested that lemon garlic may be an effective alternative to NAOCL. [130] Garlic extract is biocompatible and has shown strong antibacterial activity. However, its odour, unpleasant taste and short shelf life pose a problem when used in the oral environment. The authors have suggested the addition of flavourings to make the taste more pleasant for the patient. [108]

❖ **Grape seed extract (Vitis Vinifera) :**

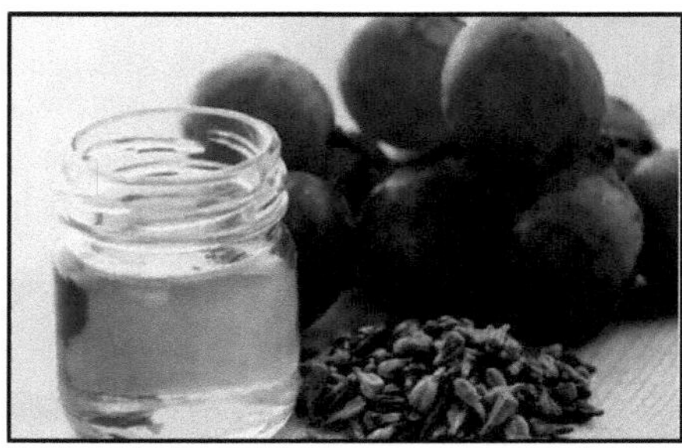

Figure 27: Grape seed oil [177].

Grapes are one of the most widely consumed fruits in the world **(Figure 27).** It is a rich source of polyphenols, carbohydrates and fruit acids. The presence of phenolic compounds in grape seeds gives it a significant therapeutic effect.The proanthocyanidins (PA) present in grape seeds strengthen the collagen fibres of the dentinal tubules and improve the mechanical properties of the tooth structure. They are also known for their anti-oxidant, anti-inflammatory and antibacterial properties. [23] Several authors have compared NaOCl and grape seed extract as endodontic irrigants.Cechin et al in 2015 observed that 6.5% grape seed extract had greater antimicrobial activity than 2.5% NaOCL and resulted in improved mechanical properties of the dentinal walls unlike NaOCL which reduced flexural, tensile and fracture strength. [23,40]

Moreover, it has been reported in the literature that grape seed extract as an irrigant produces complex bonds with the dentin collagen matrix, which improves root canal obturation, whereas grape seed extract as an irrigant produces complex bonds with the dentin collagen matrix, which improves root canal obturation. NAOCL promotes structural changes in the inorganic and organic components of dentine, in particular collagen, thus increasing the risk of fracture, particularly in the thin walls. [23,40] Margono et al in 2017 investigated the ability of grape seed extract obtained by maceration at different concentrations to remove dentin smear layer in the apical third. The results indicated that the dentin smear removal potential of grape seed extract was satisfactory but slightly lower than 17% EDTA and independent of concentration. [91]

Soligo et al in 2018 revealed that 50% grape seed extract was as effective as 6% NaOCL in reducing bacteria from E.faecalis infected ducts. [136] Proanthocyanidins damage microbial cells by altering the selective permeability of the membrane, leading to leakage of essential intracellular substances. [23] Similarly, Fallios et al in 2019 evaluated the antimicrobial efficacy of grape seed extract at 6.5% on an E. Faecalis biofilm using confocal laser scanning microscopy (CLSM) compared to NAOCL at 5.25% and CHX at 2%. The grape seed extract showed a significantly higher proportion of dead bacteria than the 2% CHX group **(Figure 28)** [51]. LBCM images of the CHX (2%) revealed that after 10 min of contact with the biofilm, only the superficial layers were slightly affected by the irrigant, while the deeper layers showed a living bacterial biofilm. This reveals a limited antibiofilm action of CHX.

(**Figure 29**) [51] Nevertheless, the NaOCL group (5.25%) showed the highest number of dead cells2. The ability of NaOCL to dissolve organic matter and attack the extracellular matrix of the biofilm explains the results obtained. (**Figure 30**) [51]

Figure 28: LBCM image of dentine disc infected with E. Faecalis biofilm 21 days after exposure to grape seed extract (6.5%). [51]

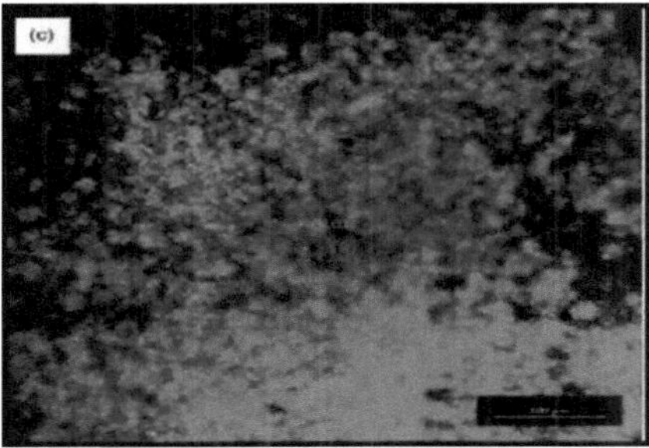

Figure 29: LBCM image of dentine disc infected with E. Faecalis biofilm 21 days after exposure to CHX (2%). [51]

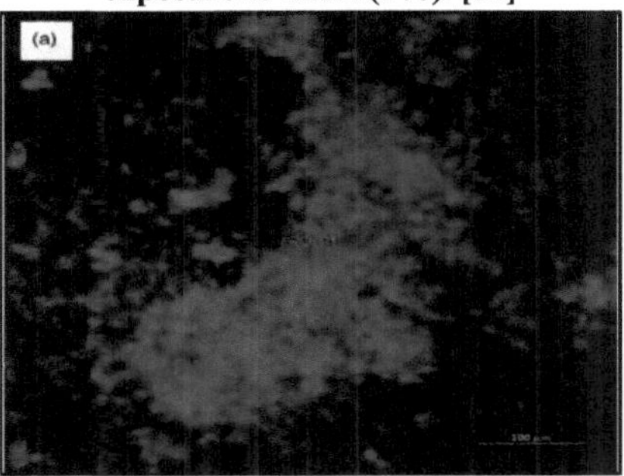

Figure 30: MCBL image of dentine disc infected with E. Faecalis biofilm 21 days after exposure to NAOCL (5.25%). [51]

Although this natural product appears to be a promising endodontic irrigant, it does not fulfil all the criteria for being a clinically effective endodontic irrigant. Therefore, further studies are needed to evaluate its ability to penetrate deep dentinal tubules, its bactericidal activity against different species of the root canal system and the possibility of tooth staining. [23]

❖ Turmeric (Curcuma Longa)

Curcumin (diferuloylmethane), turmeric's main natural polyphenol, is known for its anti-inflammatory, antioxidant, antimicrobial and anticancer activity. [8] Curcumin's antimicrobial capacity is attributed to its ability to damage the bacterial cell membrane and inhibit cell proliferation. [94]

According to Praveenkumar et al in 2013, curcumin in an in vitro model proved effective against the following bacteria: Streptococcus mutans, Actinomyces viscosus, Lactobacillus casei, Porphyromonas gingivalis and Prevotella intermedia. [147]

Combined with photodynamic therapy, the aqueous preparation of turmeric revealed a toxic effect against gram (+) and gram (-) bacteria (Haukviv et al in 2010). [33] According to an in vitro study conducted by Neelakantan et al in 2013 on extracted human teeth, curcumin was shown to have similar efficacy to NaOCl (3%) in eradicating E.faecalis biofilm and superior to CHX (2%). [33]

Similarly, Neelakantan et al in 2015 observed that photoactivated curcumin had the ability to remove E. faecalis biofilm from the walls of the root canal.[103] The ability of photoactivated curcumin to remove E. faecalis biofilm from the walls of the root canal was also observed. A curcumin solution activated by blue light also proved to be a better disinfectant against E. Faecalis in both its planktonic and biofilm forms. In addition, curcumin showed no toxicity against odontoblast-like cells, undifferentiated pulp cells and human embryonic stem cells. [147] The major advantages of curcumin are its availability, cost-effectiveness, increased shelf-life and low toxicity. However, to date, all published studies evaluating its effect on endodontic bacteria have been in vitro, and its effectiveness in vivo remains to be determined. [8]

❖ Clove (Syzygium aromaticum) :

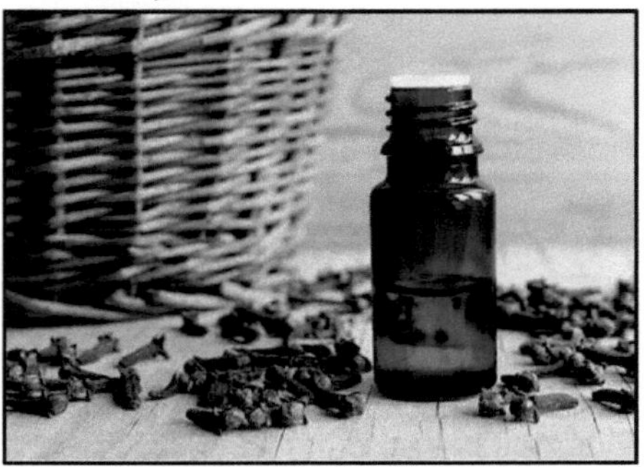

Figure 31:Oil extracted from clove [158].

Cloves are the aromatic dried flower buds of a tree in the Myrtaceae family of the genus Syzygium aromaticum **(Figure 31)**. [61]

Clove has long been used in dentistry for its analgesic, antifungal, antimicrobial and anti-inflammatory properties. [124]

The essential oils in cloves are eugenol, isoeugenol and vanillin, which have antioxidant and antibacterial effects. [33] Eugenol, the active ingredient in cloves, has a sedative effect on pulp inflammation, which is why it is used as an inter-session medication in a well wrung-out cotton ball (in cases of irreversible pulp inflammation) in everyday practice.

Zinc oxide has also been combined with zinc oxide to form a paste with different applications:

• Temporary crown filling

• Cavity floor

• Pulpotomy

• Root canal cement

• Prosthetic cement

• Antiseptic dressing in case of dry alveolitis. [124]

Eugenol acts on bacteria by sensitising the phospholipid bilayer of the microbial cytoplasmic membrane, leading to bacterial cell death. [37] Gupta et al in 2013 studied the antibacterial efficacy of different concentrations of ethanolic ethanolic extracts of Ocimum   sanctum (Tulsi), Cinnamomum zeylanicum (cinnamon) and Syzygium aromaticum (clove) against E.faecalis at different time intervals. The diffusion test in agar wells, the micro-dilution test and the biofilm sensitivity test on cellulose nitrate membrane and in a tooth model were used. Extracts of O. sanctum, C. zeylanicum and S. aromaticum showed antimicrobial effects against E. faecalis in both planktonic and biofilm forms, but NaOCL (3%) was the most effective of all the groups. [61] A similar study published by Gupta et al in 2016 found that Syzygium aromaticum and Cinnamomum zeylanicum showed an intracanal bacterial reduction of Enterococcus faecalis of 80-85% while O. Sanctum showed only a 70-75% reduction. In contrast, NaOCl (3%) showed a bacterial reduction of 96-100%. [63]Similarly, these three plant extracts were selected to study their ability to eliminate the dentin smear layer compared with 3% NaOCL combined with 17% EDTA. SEM observations revealed that these were effective in cleaning root canal walls only when combined with EDTA (17%) with maximum activity of S. Aromaticum extract combined with EDTA. **(Figure 32)**[60].

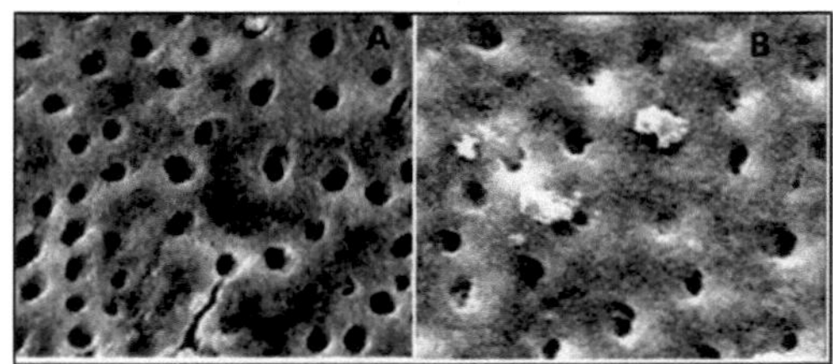

Figure 32:(A): SEM view showing complete removal of dentin sludge (NaOCL+EDTA); (B): SEM view showing partial removal of dentin sludge (S. aromaticum +EDTA) (Magnification*1500) [60].

❖ **Cinnamon (Cinnamomum zeylanicum) :**

Ceylon cinnamon (Cinnamomum zeylanicum or verum) is a species of tree in the Lauraceae family **(Figure 33)**. Cinnamon oil obtained from the leaves and root bark has antioxidant, antimutagenic and antimicrobial activity, mainly due to the presence of cinnamaldehyde, the most active component. [89]

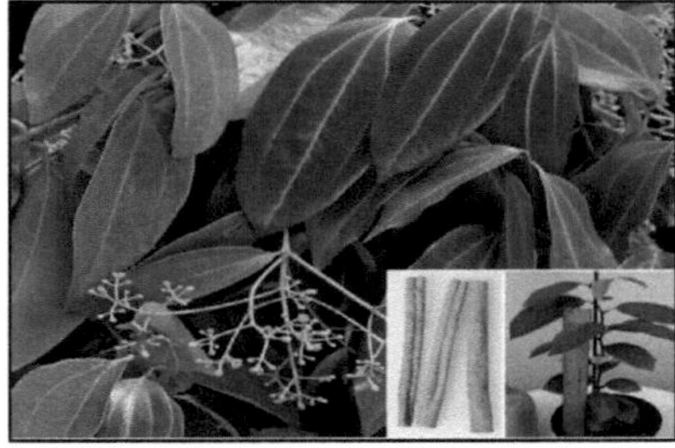

Figure 33: Cinnamon leaves [170].

Cinnamaldehyde causes the death of microbial cells by inhibiting the activity of amino acid decarboxylation in the cell, resulting in energy deprivation. [89]

When ethanolic extract of cinnamon was evaluated as an endodontic irrigant on human teeth, it showed maximum efficacy against Candida albicans and minimal efficacy against E.Faecalis, which is superior to turmeric but inferior to garlic. [108]

This result is in line with a study carried out by Bardaji et al in 2015 which revealed that cinnamon essential oil did not inhibit the growth of E. Faecalis. However, it had shown moderate activity against Fusobacterium nucleatum, Actinomyces naeslundii, Prevotella nigrescens and Streptococcus mutans. [30] On their part, Ala Mahdi et al in 2018 studied the antimicrobial activity of ethanolic extract of cinnamon (EEC) against clinical isolates of oral pathogens (Enterococcus faecalis, Candida albicans, Staphylococcus aureus, Pseudomonas aeruginosa and Streptococcus mutans) in comparison with 5.25% NaOCl. [86]

They found satisfactory antibacterial activity of 25% cinnamon extract compared with 5.25% NAOCL for all the bacteria tested, except for Staphylococcus aureus, where NAOCL produced a wider zone of inhibition, demonstrating its effectiveness. A study carried out by

Eve Marcoux et al in 2019 evaluated the effect of nisin, cinnamon essential oil and three polyphenols derived from liquorice (licochalcone A, licoricidin and glabridin) on the survival of E. Faecalis, in planktonic form or organised in a biofilm. All the compounds tested resulted in a reduction in biofilm formation in proportion to the reduction in bacterial growth. In particular, cinnamon essential oil which proved to be the most potent bacteriostatic agent with a minimum inhibitory concentration (MIC) between 1.56 and 3.13 µg/mL and a bactericidal agent against E.faecalis at a minimum bactericidal concentration (MBC) of 12.5 µg/mL. [90] To assess their biocompatibility, the authors tested the effects of the products used on different cell lines: stem cells from the apical papilla (SCAP), oral epithelial cells (B11) and gingival fibroblasts (HGF- 1).They observed no significant cytotoxic effect of polyphenols or nisin at concentrations effective against E.Faecalis.As for cinnamon essential oil, it appears to have a cytotoxic effect when used at concentrations greater than 0.39 µg /mL. [90]

❖ Tea tree oil (Melaleuca alternifolia) :

Tea tree (Melaleuca alternifolia) is an Australian tree from the Myrtaceae family with powerful antifungal and antimicrobial properties **(Figure 34)**.

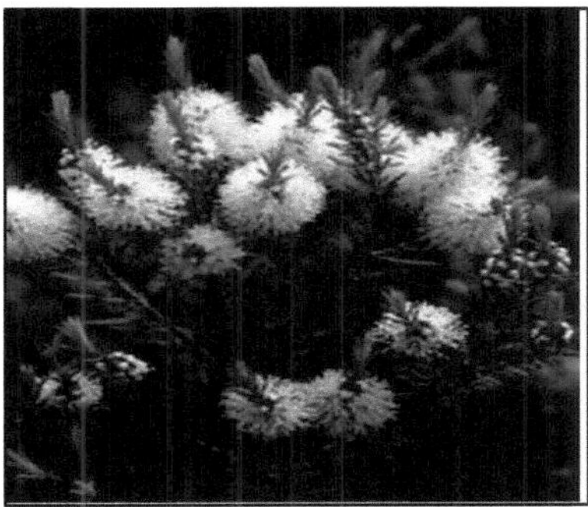

Figure 34: Tea tree flowers [34].

According to Neelakantan et al in 2011, tea tree oil extracted from the leaves of Melaleuca alternifolia has a mild solvating action that could be useful in dissolving necrotic pulp tissue. [33]

Terpinen-4-ol, a major component of tea tree oil, acts on the bacterial cell wall by affecting the permeability of the cell membrane, thereby preventing bacterial growth. [100] According to a study evaluating the antibacterial efficacy of tea tree oil, 3% sodium hypochlorite and 2% Chlorhexidine against E faecalis using the agar well diffusion method, tea tree oil showed comparable inhibition of bacterial growth to sodium hypochlorite and CHX.[80] The study also found that tea tree oil was more effective than CHX in inhibiting bacterial growth. Tea tree oil was extracted from the leaves of Melaleuca alternifolia by distillation and then prepared to be miscible i n 85% ethanol at 200°C. to obtain a concentration of 2% by volume. The concentration recommended in the literature is 2.5% to 5%, which guarantees antibacterial power without toxic effects. [80]

These results are consistent with another study conducted by Sinha et al in 2015 where 2% tea tree oil showed significant antimicrobial activity against E faecalis however lower than CHX 2% and NaOCL (5%). [134] Jianyan Qi et al in 2021 evaluated the effect of tea tree oil on E faecalis biofilm using scanning electron microscopy (SEM) and confocal laser scanning microscopy (CLSM). The minimum inhibitory concentration (MIC) and minimum bactericidal concentration (MBC) were 0.25% and 0.5% respectively, and the bacterial inhibition rate and destruction time were dose-dependent. The study revealed that tea tree oil was able to inhibit E faecalis by destroying the cell membrane. SEM and LBCM images showed that this oil could reduce bacterial aggregation, biofilm thickness and inhibit biofilm formation. The authors concluded that tea tree oil has the potential to be effective against E. faecalis infections. [116] As tea tree oil is easy to extract and cost-effective, these studies open up new avenues for the use of plant-based products as root canal irrigants or medicines.

It is essential to develop other studies with a high level of scientific evidence evaluating the toxicity of tea tree oil and its biocompatibility before recommending its clinical use. [80]

❖ **Miswak (Salvadora Persica) :**

Miswak is a traditional chewing stick made from the Miswak plant. Salvadora persica **(Figure 35)**. It has been used by the Babylonians for around seven thousand years to clean teeth and is still used by some people around the world, particularly in Africa, South America, Asia and the Middle East.

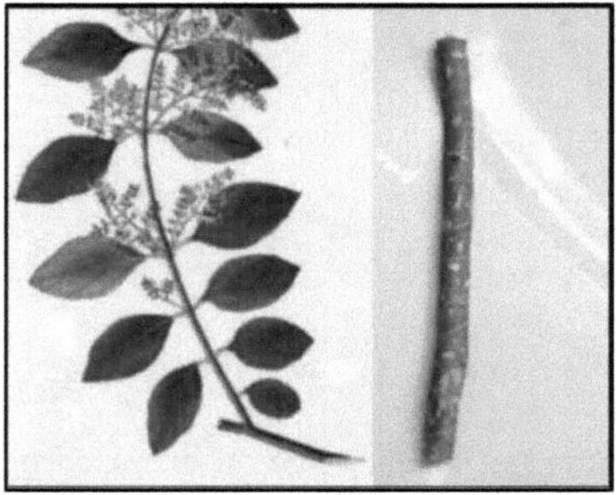

Figure 35: Leaves and roots of Miswak (Salvadora persica) [13].

It contains several bioactive ingredients. The most important and effective ingredient is benzyl isothiocyanate, a major antimicrobial volatile oil. The calcium, chloride and fluoride present in Miswak have anti-cariogenic properties and prevent tartar formation and tooth demineralisation. Vitamin C also helps heal and repair oral tissues and acts as an antioxidant. [5] Several studies have reported the effectiveness of Meswak in controlling dental plaque and preventing caries when used as a toothbrush, in toothpastes or as a mouthwash. [153] In addition, authors have suggested that S. persica paste can be used as an alternative material for tooth whitening that can eliminate extrinsic discolouration. This is linked to the presence of crystals in the Miswak, as revealed by the energy-dispersive X-ray spectroscopy technique. Thus, the latter can act as a natural abrasive. [153]

Other studies have evaluated the use of Miswak extract for root canal irrigation.

Al-Sabawi et al in 2007 compared the antimicrobial activity of S. persica, sodium hypochlorite, chlorhexidine and normal saline in vitro. The results of this study showed that 15% alcoholic extract of Salvadora Persica, 5.25% NaOCL solution, and 0.2% CHX had a significant antimicrobial effect against aerobic and anaerobic bacteria recovered from teeth with necrotic pulps, while normal saline had no significant antimicrobial effect. [20]

However, a recent study in 2022 evaluating 10 mg/ml SP ethanolic extract as an endodontic irrigant compared with 1% NaOCL revealed that SP ethanolic extract showed significantly weaker cytotoxic and antimicrobial effects than NaOCl exposure[17].

As well as being antibacterial, an endodontic irrigant must be biocompatible. The authors therefore conducted a study to evaluate the effect of aqueous and ethanolic extracts of Salvadora persica at different concentrations on the proliferation and viability of human dental pulp stem cells. The results showed that high concentrations of ethanolic extracts of SP (1.43-5.75-mg/ml) were cytotoxic on human dental pulp stem cells while aqueous extract of SP at certain concentrations (0.08 to 1.43 mg/ml) could promote cell proliferation[97]. Salvadora persica extract was also recommended as an intracanal medicament because it showed better antibacterial effects against E. faecalis and S. mutans on days 3 and 7 than calcium hydroxide. [5, 27]

❖ German chamomile (Matricaria recutita) :

German chamomile (Matricaria recutita) is a medicinal plant native to Europe and Western Asia, generally taken orally as an infusion **(Figure 36)**.It has an antibacterial, anti-inflammatory, antifungal and analgesic effect and is able to inhibit infections of the oral cavity making it an ideal component for mouthwashes. [143]

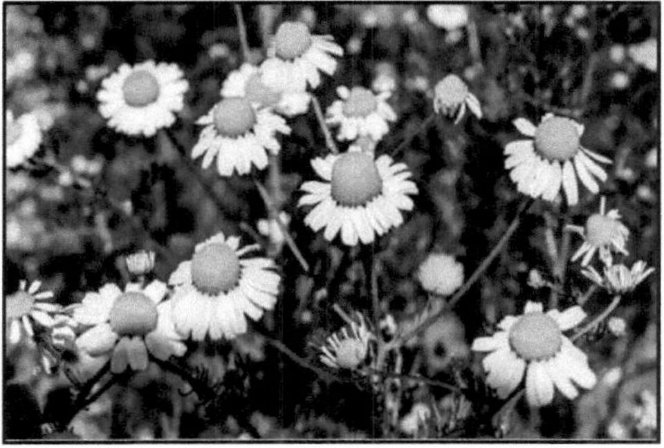

Figure 36: German chamomile flowers [166].

In a study evaluating the efficacy of hydroalcoholic extract of chamomile in endodontic irrigation, it was found that chamomile was more effective than 2.5% NaOCL in removing dentinal sludge but less effective than sodium hypochlorite combined with EDTA. [146]

This result is in agreement with a previous study by Sadr Lahijani et al in 2006. [8] The elimination of dentinal sludge could be explained by the presence of acid components such as caprylic acid, chlorogenic acid, o- caumaric acid and dihydroxybenzoic acid in the extract. [146]Another study conducted by J. Sowjanyaa et al in 2017 by SEM analysis showed that chamomile did not show satisfactory results in terms of dentin sludge removal compared to EDTA 17% **(Figure 37).** [140]

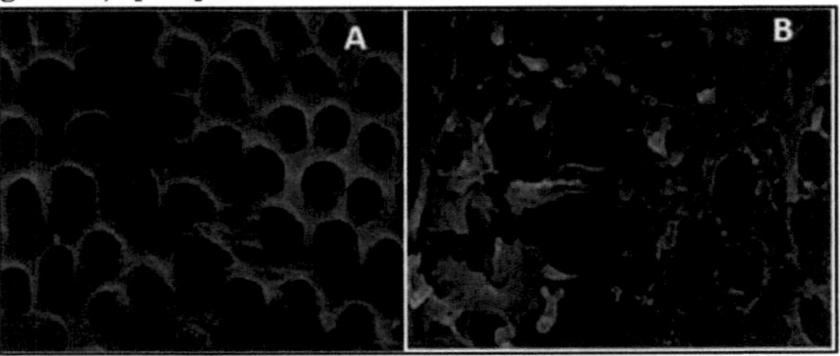

Figure 37: SEM observation Magnification (*2000)

(A): EDTA group; (B) Chamomile group [140].

❖ **Passion fruit (Passiflora edulis) :**

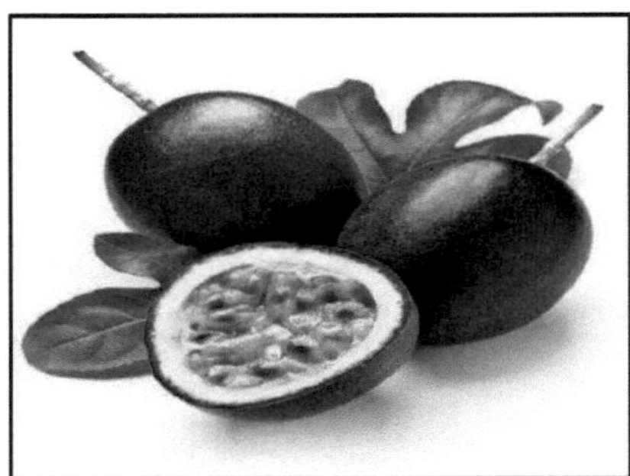

Figure 38: Passion fruit [175]

It is a climbing plant that belongs to the Passifloraceae family and grows in tropical regions (Figure 38). It is widely used in folk medicine in South America. The constituents of the various extracts include flavonoids, alkaloids, cyanogenic compounds, glycosides, vitamins, minerals and terpenoid compounds. [147]This plant has antibacterial, antifungal, antihypertensive and anti-inflammatory properties. [147] Passion fruit pulp extract has been shown to be effective against mutans streptococci at a concentration of 40 to 45%. [132] According to an in vitro study evaluating the antimicrobial capacity of different concentrations of passion fruit extract compared with saline solution and NaOCl against E. faecalis, the 20% and 30% alcoholic passion fruit extract significantly reduced the bacterial load. Nevertheless, passion fruit extract at 30% had a significant antimicrobial effect against E faecalis comparable to 5.25% NaOCL. [54]Similarly, Jayahari et al in 2014 evaluated the efficacy of different concentrations of aqueous and alcoholic passion fruit juice extracts in removing E. Faecalis compared to NaOCL. The extracts were prepared using a cold maceration technique.The broth dilution test revealed negative growth of E. Faecalis by the 20% alcoholic extract at 30 min, the 20% aqueous extract at 1 h, NaOCl 2.5% at 10 min and NaOCl 5.25% at 1 min. In conclusion, NaOCl showed better antibacterial efficacy than passion fruit extracts. [76]There is insufficient in vitro research evaluating the efficacy of passion fruit as a root canal irrigant. Other studies are therefore to assess the safety and biocompatibility of passion fruit extract as an irrigant before recommending it for clinical use.

❖ Guava (Psidium Guajava) :

The guava (Psidium Guajava) is a species of fruit tree in the Myrtaceae family, native to tropical America **(Figure 39)**. It is a plant rich in tannins, phenols, triterpenes, flavonoids, essential oils, saponins, carotenoids, lectins, vitamins and fatty acids. It has anti-inflammatory, antimicrobial, antioxidant and antimutagenic properties. In addition, its leaves are rich in Guajaverin, a plant flavonoid that inhibits the formation of S. mutans and S. aureus. [143,154]

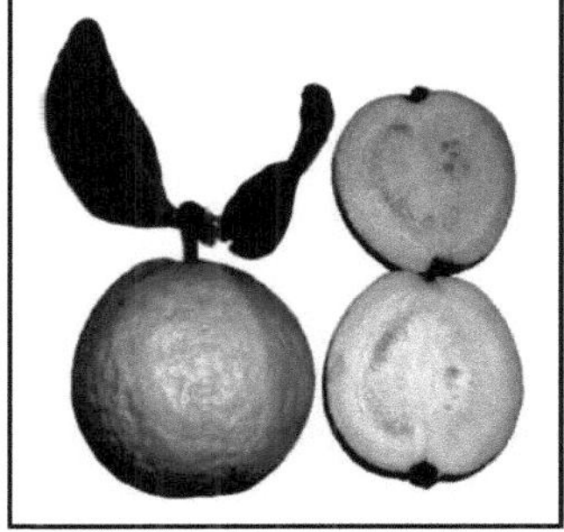

Figure 39: Guava fruit [187].

Authors have reported the in vitro efficacy of the ethanolic extract of guava leaves against Streptococcus mutans (S. mutans) and Enterococcus faecalis (E. faecalis). [101]The tannins present in guava leaves are polyphenolic compounds that interfere with protein synthesis, thus exerting antibacterial activity. Flavonoids form complexes with extracellular proteins that are soluble in the bacterial cell wall. [101] In addition, it has been reported that an ethanol extract from Psidium guajava at 20% has a very high antimicrobial activity against E. Faecalis that is similar to 2% Chlorhexidine. [114]

Guava leaf extract at different concentrations showed little or no cytotoxic effect and high antibacterial activity against E.Faecalis but lower than NaOCL (2.5%) [73]. According to a study conducted by Dubey Sandeep in 2015 evaluating the antibacterial effect of herbal alternatives (Emblica officinalis, Psidium Guajava), BioPure MTAD and 2.5% sodium hypochlorite against E.faecalis, it was shown that BioPure MTAD has the highest efficacy.[47] It has also been concluded that Emblica officinalis and Psidium guajava are effective antibacterial agents against E. Faecalis and can be used to reduce root canal microflora. [47]

❖ **Gum Ferula (Férula Gummosa) :**

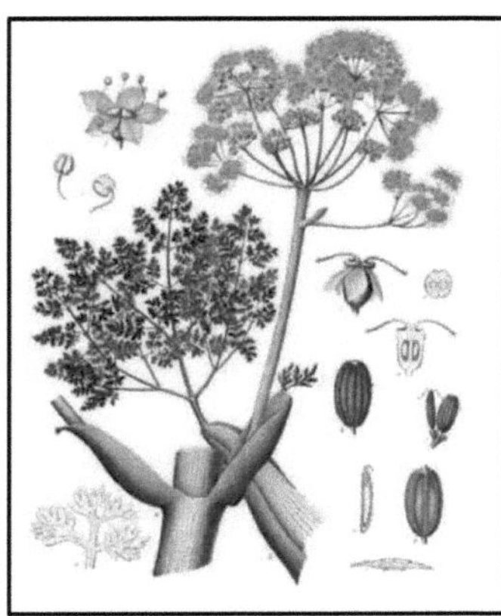

Figure 40: Ferula gummosa [183].

Gumweed is a herbaceous perennial plant of the Apiaceae family that grows widely in Central Asia, the Mediterranean region and elsewhere in the world. and North Africa **(Figure 40).** The plant has been shown to possess favourable antimicrobial, anti-nociceptive, anti-inflammatory, anticonvulsant, antioxidant and antispasmodic activities. [147]

A study by Ghasemi et al in 2005 showed that the essential oil (EO) of Ferula gummosa (FG) had strong antimicrobial activity against Gram (+) and Gram (-) bacteria and also against candida albicans. [56]Later in 2015, Abbaszadegan et al compared the antimicrobial efficacy of Ferula gummosa EO against E. Faecalis, Streptococcus mitis, Staphylococcus aureus and Candida albicans compared to NaOCl 5% and CHX 0.2%. [3] Hydro distillation of Ferula gummosa fruits gave an excellent EO yield of 32%. Gas chromatography/mass spectrometry (GC/MS) was used to determine the chemical compositions of the oil, 27 constituents were recognised by this technique of which the major component of the oil was p-pinene (51.83%) and the minor components were a- pinene, 83-carene, p-phellandrene and carvacrol methyl ether.The authors concluded that Ferula Gummosa EO is a biocompatible agent with potent antimicrobial potential when used as a root canal disinfectant. Nevertheless, further studies are needed to assess its efficacy on bacterial biofilms present in the root canal. [3]

❖ **Carvacrol :**

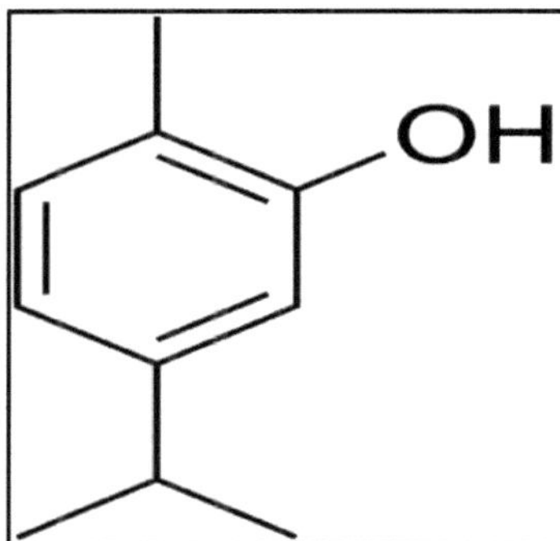

Figure 41: Chemical formula of Carvacrol [180].

Carvacrol (2-methyl-5-isopropylphenol) is a monoterpene phenol that occurs as a thick oil that gives off a warm, pungent odour characteristic of oregano **(Figure 41)**. [180]Carvacrol is obtained from oregano (origanum vulgare), thyme (thymus vulgaris), watercress and monarda. It is commercially available from various companies such as Sigma Aldrich, Biocore, MP Biochemicals, Life Chemicals &Glentham Life Sciences Ltd [135].

This plant extract is used as a food additive approved by the Food and Drug Administration (FDA) (FDA reg. No 172.5151) to prevent bacterial contamination. [104]

It inhibits the growth of several strains of bacteria, such as Escherichia coli, Bacillus cereus and Pseudomonas aeruginosa. It works by disrupting the cell membrane. In addition, it has antifungal activity against Candida albicans in root canals comparable to 5.25% NaOCL. [1]

The study by Nasrat et al in 2009 revealed that carvacrol has an anti-inflammatory action and when used as an endodontic irrigant at a At a concentration of 0.6%, it was able to eliminate 99% of the bacteria (E. faecalis) in 5 minutes. [104] Carvacrol has also been recommended as an intracanal medication, as it has been shown to be as effective as calcium hydroxide in eliminating Enterococcus faecalis. [6] That said, further studies with a high level of scientific evidence are needed before its use in clinical practice can be approved.

■**Other plant extracts**

Myrtle (Myrtus communis), nutmeg (Myristica fragrans), lemon solution and Jieeryin solution have also been briefly described in the literature as natural alternatives for irrigating and disinfecting root canals.

❖ **Myrtle: (Myrtus communis)** belongs to the Myrtaceae family and is distributed around tropical regions **(Figure 42).**

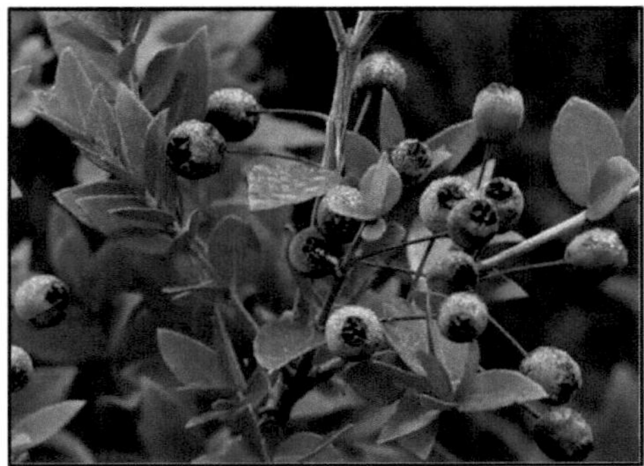

Figure 42: Myrtle plant [168].

Compared with NaOCL (5%) and CHX (2%), the essential oil extracted from the leaves of M. communis with an MIC of between 0.032 and 32 µg/mL was an antimicrobial agent effective against persistent endodontic micro-organisms (E. faecalis, S. aureus and C. albicans). [33] Raja Sulieman in 2009 evaluated the antibacterial effect of alcoholic extract of Myrtus communis when used as an endodontic irrigant, the results revealed a significant antibacterial effect at different concentrations in particular at 35%, comparable to 5.25% NaOCL. [8]

❖ **Nutmeg (Myristica fragrans) :**

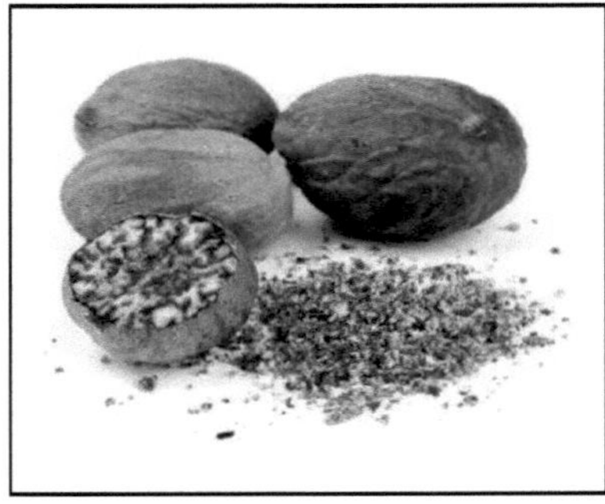

Figure 43: Nutmeg [173]

Vinothkumar et al in 2013 evaluated different plant extracts as endodontic irrigants against Enterococcus faecalis and Candida albicans using real-time quantitative polymerase chain reaction (PCR). The efficacy of the extracts in descending order was as follows: Azadirachta indica, Curcuma longa, Myristica fragrans, Terminalia Chebula and Aloe vera. [8] Furthermore, according to a study by Setty et al in 2020 evaluating the antimicrobial effect of Myristica fragrans essential oil on endodontic pathogens involved in primary apical periodontitis (Escherichia coli, Staphylococcus aureus, Enterococcus faecalis, Streptococcus mutans, Candida albicans, Lactobacillus casei, Actinomyces viscosus, Prevotella intermedia and Porphyromonas gingivalis), the essential oil of M. fragrans was extracted by hydrodistillation and proved effective against all the endodontic micro-organisms tested.

The active components of nutmeg essential oil are myristicin, myristic acid, trimyristin, elemicin and safrole. Its antibacterial activity is attributed mainly to myristic acid. [127]

❖ **Lemon solution :**

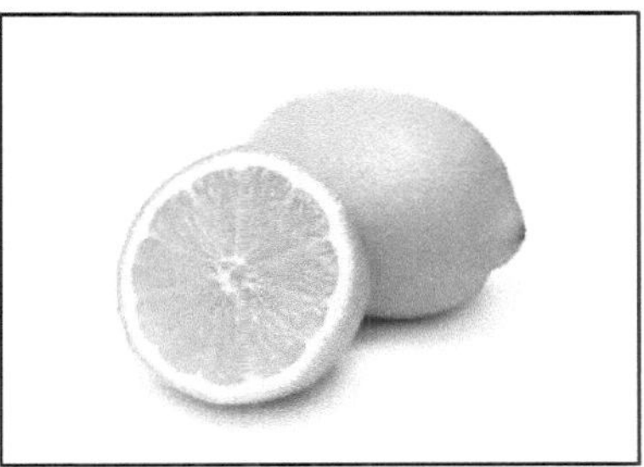

Figure 44: Lemon [164]

Lemon solution (pH=2.21) is a natural source of citric acid (pH=1.68) which acts as a chelating agent with less acidity (Figure 44). [99]Lemon has been proposed as an intracanal medicament due to its high antibacterial action against E.faecalis, however its biological behaviour on periapical tissue needs to be evaluated. (Sawsan T et al ,2004). [135]

❖ **Jieeryin's solution:**

A Chinese herbal preparation. [33] Thanks to its detoxifying and anti-inflammatory properties, 30% jieeryin solution used in combination with ultrasound has been proposed as an alternative to sodium hypochlorite in root canal irrigation. [8]

3. Intra- root canal medication

To complement the action of the chemo-mechanical preparation, antibacterial products are inserted into the root canals for additional disinfection.Calcium hydroxide in paste form has always been considered a reference material for intracanal medication. $Ca(OH)_2$ is a broad-spectrum alkaline and antiseptic agent. It acts by denaturing bacterial plasma membrane proteins through the action of hydroxyl ions. However, it is not without its limitations. Calcium hydroxide is not effective against all the pathogenic microbes present in the root canal, such as Enterococcus faecalis and candidas albicans, which are implicated in endodontic failure. [143,128]E.faecalis has the ability to resist the alkaline environment produced by calcium hydroxide. It has a proton pump that actively pumps hydrogen ions to neutralise the alkaline environment and maintain a constant cytoplasmic PH. [90] In addition, $Ca(OH)2$ when placed for longer than 4 weeks in apexification procedures reduces the microhardness of dentin making it prone to fracture. [128] Taking into account the limitations of the chemicals currently used in endodontic practice as intracanal medication, several natural materials and their derivatives have been tested as future alternatives for this indication. [128]

❖ **Casearia sylvestris Swartz :**

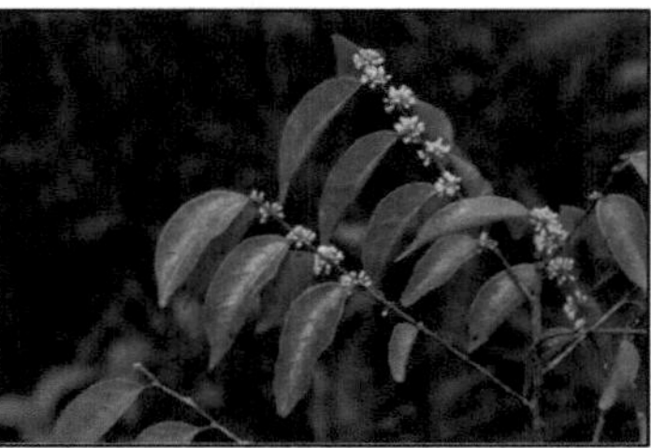

Figure 45: Casearia sylvestris Swartz [165]

Casearia sylvestris Swartz is a medicinal plant of the Salicaceae family found in tropical America and Brazil. It has anti-inflammatory and antimicrobial activity. [80]Indeed, the alcoholic extract of C. sylvestris acts on the acute phase of inflammation by inhibiting phospholipase A2, a pro-inflammatory enzyme. [131]Given its anti-inflammatory effect observed in animal models, Da silva et al in 2004 suggested that this plant could be a good alternative as an intracanal drug. Thus, in-depth studies are needed on this subject. [131]

In 2017, Cavenago et al added propylene glycol extracts from Casearia sylvestris to MTA and observed an increase in the antimicrobial effect with an increase in its setting time without hindering the biocompatibility of MTA. [33]

❖ **Papain :**

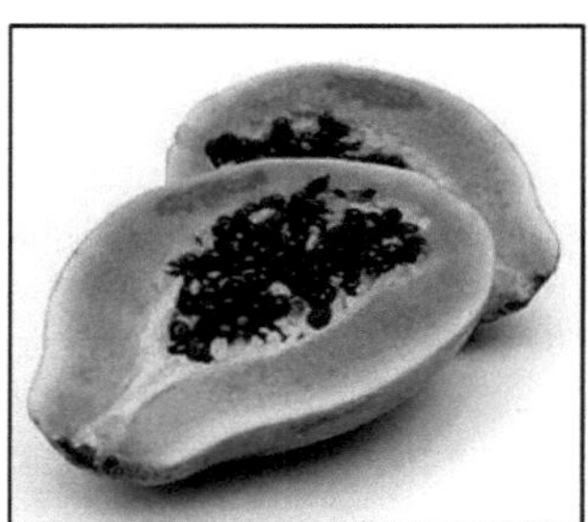

Figure 46: Papaya fruit [172].

Papain is a proteolytic enzyme extracted from the latex between the papaya peel and pulp. It has significant antibacterial and anti-inflammatory properties. [35] Papain gel has been proposed as an irrigation solution because of its bactericidal power against E. Faecalis and its ability to dissolve pulp tissue, unlike CHX. [112]Bhardwaj et al in 2012 studied the antimicrobial efficacy of natural extracts in the form of gels of M. citrifolia, papain, A.Vera, 2% CHX and calcium hydroxide in the disinfection of dentinal tubules contaminated with E.faecalis.M. citrifolia gel (86.2%) showed better antimicrobial efficacy than aloe vera gel (78.9%), papain gel (67.3%) and calcium hydroxide (64.3%). However, chlorhexidine gel (2%) showed maximum antimicrobial activity against E. faecalis. [35]

❖ **Morinda citrifolia :**

Morinda citrifolia has also been studied as an intracanal medication. The antimicrobial activity of 2% CHX gel, propolis, Morinda citrifolia juice and calcium hydroxide was evaluated on root canal dentin infected with E. faecalis at two different depths (200 μm and 400 μm) and at three time intervals (day 1, 3 and 5).It was concluded that propolis and Morinda Citrifolia were effective against E. Faecalis in the dentine of extracted teeth. [81]
In another in vitro study conducted by Prabhakar et al in 2013, Morinda Citrifolia was compared with Chlorhexidine. The authors found that Morinda Citrifolia had significant antibacterial activity but less than 0.2% Chlorhexidine after 28 days. The authors attributed this antibacterial activity to the presence of Alizarin, Scopoletin, Acubin and Asperuloside. [8]This result is consistent with the study by Bhardwaj et al in 2012 who found that 2% CHX gel showed 100% inhibition against E faecalis at depths of 200 and 400 μm from day 1 to day 5 compared to 86.2% for Morinda Citrifolia gel. The efficacy of M. Citrifolia gel remained the same over the 5-day period. [35]

❖ **Tulsi (Ocimum Sanctum or Ocimum tenuiflorum) :**

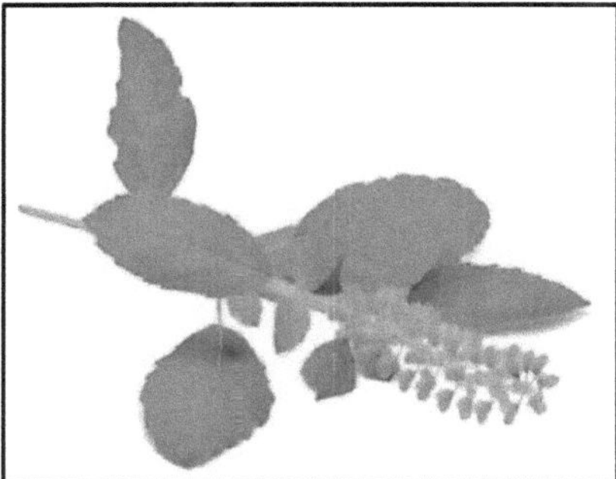

Figure 47: Tulsi leaves [161].

Ocimum Sanctum or Ocimum tenuiflorum, also known as tulsi basil or sweet basil, is a herbaceous plant of the Lamiaceae family widely grown in India. In addition to its antibacterial properties, Tulsi is anti-inflammatory, highly biocompatible and non-toxic. [128]

The antibacterial effect of Tulsi is associated with the presence of linoleic acid, eugenol, carvacrol and linolenic acid. [41]

Moreover, several in vitro studies have found that Tulsi extract had remarkable antimicrobial activity against E. Faecalis in comparison with 2% chlorhexidine (Gupta et al. 2013, Chandrappa et al. 2015). [128, 41] However, an in vivo study carried out by Goldy Rathee et al in 2020 revealed that Tulsi and Neem extracts had a significant antimicrobial effect in primary endodontic infections compared with 2% CHX. Consequently, the authors recommended their use in intracanal irrigation and medication. [96]

* **Propolis :**

Several in vitro studies have evaluated the use of propolis as an intracanal drug due to the fact that it is a biocompatible material with less cytotoxicity compared to calcium hydroxide (Al Shaher et al, 2004; Madhubala et al, 2011; Mori et al, 2014). [128] Indeed, Awawdeh et al in 2009 observed that the antimicrobial activity of 30% propolis solution against E. Faecalis species at 1 and 2 days was superior to that of calcium hydroxide[25].

In 2010, Kandaswamy et al carried out a study to evaluate the antimicrobial activity of 2% Chlorhexidine gel, propolis, propolis juice and propolis juice. Morinda citrifolia (MCJ), 2% povidone-iodine (POV-I) versus calcium hydroxide on root dentin infected with Enterococcus faecalis at two different depths (200 µm and 400 µm) and at 3 time intervals (Day 1, 3 and 5). [81]

The results of the study showed that propolis had better anti-microbial activity than Ca(OH)$_2$ and that 2% CHX performed better than propolis. [80]

In addition, an in vitro study conducted by Carbajal et al in 2012 revealed that propolis was as effective as 2% CHX gel against E.Faecalis after 14 days of application and more effective than calcium hydroxide. However, only CHX (2%) had statistically significant antifungal efficacy against C. albicans. [39]

Propolis has also been proposed as a vehicle for calcium hydroxide since it has the ability to diffuse through dentinal tubules. [29]

Aqueous, ethanolic and hydroalcoholic extracts of propolis have been shown to have analgesic and anti-inflammatory properties in the pulp by inhibiting cyclooxygenase-2 and reducing the production of pro-inflammatory cytokines responsible for pain. [151]

Therefore, Shabbir et al in 2020 conducted a clinical study to evaluate the effect of Chinese propolis paste on postoperative pain compared to calcium hydroxide (control) at different time intervals on necrotic teeth with peri-apical images. **(Figure 48)** [129]

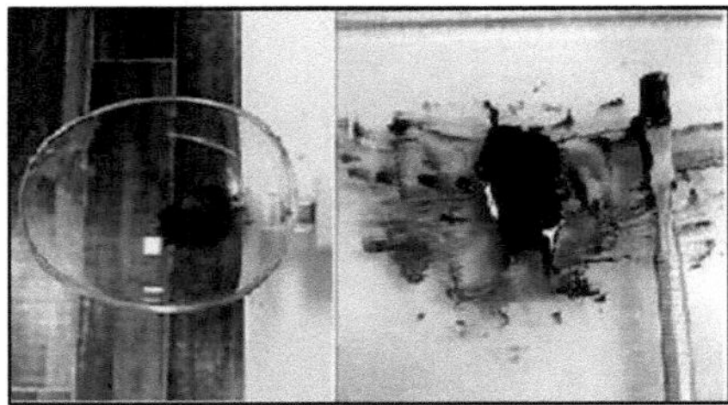

Figure 48: 200 mg of propolis powder mixed with saline solution [129].

They found that propolis was as effective as calcium hydroxide in preventing postoperative endodontic pain when used as an intracanal medication. **(Figure 49)** [129]

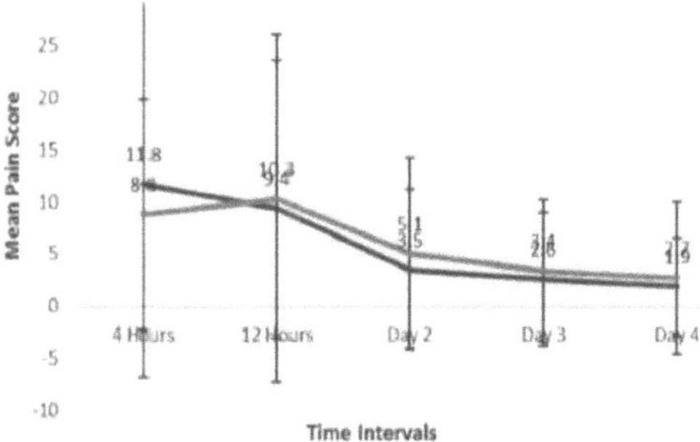

Figure 49: Pain score as a function of time [129].

❖ Azadirachta Indica (Neem)

This plant has also been suggested as an intracanal medicament.Indeed, a study evaluating the disinfection of dentinal tubules using propolis, Azadirachta Indica (alcoholic and aqueous extracts), 2% Chlorhexidine gel and calcium hydroxide $Ca(OH)_2$ against the biofilm of Candida Albicans formed on the dental substrate revealed that propolis and the alcoholic extract of Azadirachta Indica were as effective as 2% Chlorexhidine, while Candida Albicans was resistant to $Ca(OH)_2$. The presence of active constituents such as nimbidin and nimbolide contributes to the antifungal activity of Azadirachta Indica. [79]

In a study evaluating Neem as an intracanal drug, antimicrobial efficacy was identified using the agar diffusion method. The zone of inhibition against E.faecalis was greatest for the calcium hydroxide group followed by Neem extract. [118]This result was in agreement with the study by Mittal et al in 2021 where calcium hydroxide showed the highest antibacterial activity (5.3×10^4 CFU3/ml) followed by pomegranate gel (5.4×10^4 CFU/ml) then 5% Neem gel (10.2×10^4 CFU/ml) and Tulsi gel (10.2×10^4 CFU/ml). [95] Egyptian researchers have studied the antibacterial effect of two different plant extracts: Cinnamomum Zeylanicum (cinnamon) and Azadirachta Indica (Neem) compared with calcium hydroxide as an intracanal agent after chemo-mechanical disinfection. [32] The antibacterial effect was assessed using the agar diffusion test to count colony-forming units. The results revealed that cinnamon, Neem and $Ca(OH)_2$ showed similar antibacterial activity against E. Faecalis after 7 days of application. [32]The difference in results between the studies is attributed to the difference in methodology and concentrations. Although Azadirachta Indica has been suggested as an irrigant or intra-ductal medicine in vitro, it has a bitter taste that can be modified by adding sweeteners.More clinical studies on the efficacy of Neem extract are needed to test this natural product before recommending it for clinical use.

❖ Garlic (Allium sativum)

In addition to the studies that have evaluated garlic as an endodontic irrigant, some authors have studied its efficacy as an intracanal medicament. Indeed ,Eswar et al in 2013 observed that garlic extract showed better antibacterial efficacy compared to $Ca(OH)_2$ against E. Faecalis but lower than CHX at 2%. [128]

Another in vitro study by Rani et al in 2014 found that 5% garlic extract had a moderate inhibitory effect against Enterococcus faecalis and maximum antifungal activity against Candida albicans followed by 2% Chlorhexidine and then 5% Turmeric. [117]

❖ **Great burdock (Arctium lappa) :**

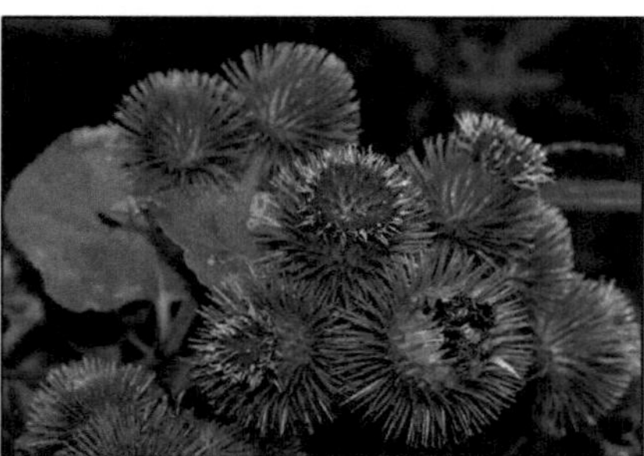

Figure 50:Great Burdock [184]

Burdock (Arctium lappa) is a plant of the Asteraceae family, widely used in folk medicine around the world for its therapeutic effects (**Figure 50**). It has antibacterial and antifungal activity, a diuretic, antioxidant and anxiolytic action, an antiplatelet aggregation effect and an HIV inhibitory action. [70]

In order to evaluate the antimicrobial potential of crude extracts of Arctium lappa leaves against microorganisms involved in endodontic infection (Enterococcus faecalis, Staphylococcus aureus, Pseudomonas aeruginosa, Bacillus subtilis and Candida albicans), Pereira et al in 2005 conducted an in vitro study which demonstrated that the constituents of Articum lappa have considerable potential for microbial inhibition against the endodontic microorganisms studied. [111] An in vitro study carried out by Tonea et al in 2006 showed that the extract of an experimental mixture of Arctium lappa root powder and Aloe vera gel was able to inhibit highly resistant micro-organisms, such as Enterococcus faecalis and Candida albicans. Specific antibiotics and antifungals were used as controls: Amoxicillin with clavulanic acid for Enterococcus faecalis and Fluconazole for Candida albicans. [144]

As endodontic bacteria are organised into biofilms, the authors stated that further studies need to be carried out to determine the behaviour of the experimental product, not only against single micro-organisms, but also against complex bacterial communities. [144]

❖ **Aloe vera gel :**

A.Vera gel has an inhibitory effect on numerous oral pathogens, in particular Streptococcus pyogenes, E. faecalis and Candida albicans. This effect has been attributed to the presence of phenolic compounds (anthraquinones). [110] According to the literature, aloe vera gel was not recommended as an intracanal irrigant, as its efficacy on E.faecalis is controversial. However, it has been used as a file lubricant during root canal shaping. [141]

In addition, it has been recommended to study the antibacterial effect of aloe vera with a longer exposure time as an intracanal drug. [123]

According to a study by Bazvand et al in 2013 which compared the antibacterial efficacy of Aloe vera, TAP tri-antibiotic paste (ciprofloxacin, metronidazole, minocycline) ,0.2% CHX gel and propolis against E.faecalis, Aloe vera showed low antibacterial activity against E.faecalis compared to the other products used. However, propolis showed similar antibacterial activity to 0.2% CHX and tri-antibiotic paste. [31]

Abbaszadegan et al in 2016 evaluated the antibacterial potential of two medicinal herbs compared to Ca(OH)$_2$ at day 1,7 and 14. The essential oils of the plants Zataria multiflora and Aloe vera showed equal antimicrobial efficacy against E. Faecalis, comparable to Ca(OH)$_2$ for the extended contact time of 14 days. [4] In the same study, carvacrol, thymol and linalool were the main constituents of both essential oils. Thymol and carvacrol are natural mono terpenes that act on the cell membrane, causing cell death, while linalool is known for its anti-inflammatory properties. [4]

According to a recent study in 2020 evaluating the efficacy of Aloe vera gel as an intracanal medication using the CFU colony-forming unit counting method, it was shown to have superior antibacterial properties to calcium hydroxide on E. Faecalis biofilm grown on extracted teeth. Indeed, aloe vera has been described in the literature as a natural antioxidant, biocompatible with periapical tissue and with significant antibacterial potential. However its effect on the physical properties of dentin and fracture resistance is unknown. [55]

❖ **Licorice (Glycyrrhiza glabra) :**

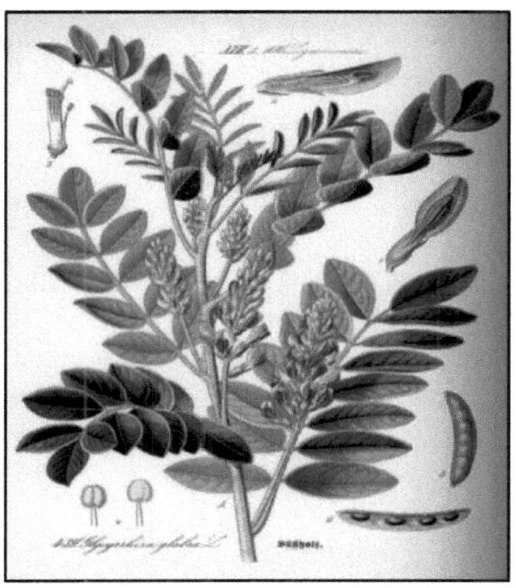

Figure 51: Licorice [188]

Licorice has antibacterial, anti-inflammatory, antiviral and anti-carcinogenic effects. [135] It has been used in the treatment of dermatitis, eczema and herpes. [147] The ethanolic extract of Licorice (Glycyrrhiza glabra) has shown strong antibacterial activity against Enterococcus faecalis, Streptococcus mutans, Actinomyces viscosus and Streptococcus sanguis. [18]Badr et al in 2010 showed that liquorice extract when used as an intracanal drug (alone or in combination with Ca(OH)$_2$ had a significant effect on E. faecalis compared to the effect obtained by Ca(OH)$_2$ alone. In addition, it was found to be biocompatible with fibroblasts and less toxic than Ca(OH)$_2$ on cells. [133,147]

❖ **Cumin (Cuminum cyminum) :**

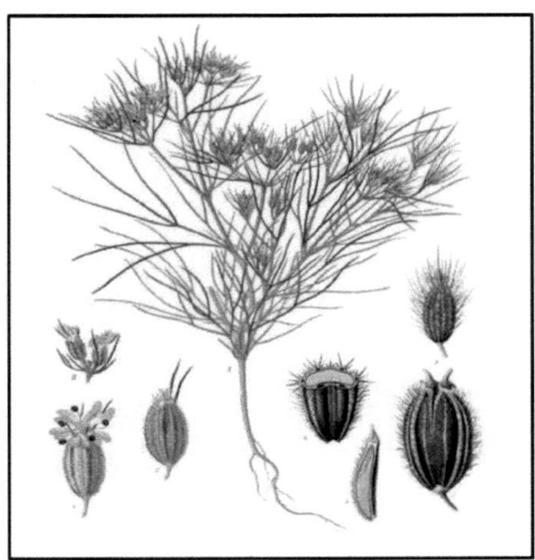

Figure 52: Cumin [182]

Cumin (Cuminum cyminum) is a herbaceous plant of the Apiaceae family found in the Mediterranean region (Figure 52).Several research studies have indicated that cumin has anti-oxidant, anti-inflammatory, analgesic and antibacterial properties. [128] Abbaszadegan et al in 2016 compared Cuminum cyminum essential oil (EO) as an intra-root canal medication versus CHX gel (2%) on planktonic and biofilm forms of bacteria isolated from teeth with persistent apical periodontitis. The results showed that C. cyminum essential oil was a more potent antimicrobial agent than CHX against all groups of micro-organisms tested (aerobic bacteria, aneorobia and E. faecalis). [2]

The antibacterial activity of the essential oil increases with time. Its mode of action depends on the chemical nature and properties of its active compounds, in particular their hydrophobic property, which allows them to penetrate the phospholipid double layer of the bacterial plasma membrane. [2]In the present study, cumin essential oil revealed 17 constituents in its composition with the predominance of cumin aldehyde and γ - terpinene, α -terpinene, β - pinene and p -cymen.In addition, the observed MIC was 14-185 µg/mL, a result that is in agreement with a previous study that reported the MIC of Tunisian cumin essential oil to be approximately 78-150 µg/mL against Gram-positive and Gram-negative microorganisms, including E. faecalis. [64]

In addition, the authors observed that cumin EO at any concentration had significantly lower toxicity than 2% CHX. However, we are unaware of the possible interactions between the chemical, physical and pharmacological properties of this oil with dentinal tubules or with root canal filling materials.

Therefore, we cannot recommend its use as an intracanal drug until further studies with a high level of scientific evidence are carried out on this subject. [2]

❖ Castor oil (Ricinus communis) :

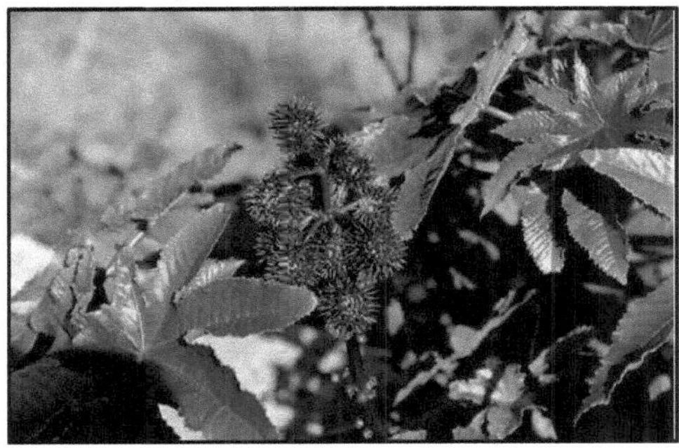

Figure 53: Ricin plant [185].

Castor oil (Ricinus communis) is a tree of tropical origin in the Euphorbiaceae family **(Figure 53)**. It has been proposed in endodontics as a drug or intracanal irrigant. [135] According to Valera et al in 2013, castor oil compared with 2.5% sodium hypchlorite and 2% chlorhexidine gel showed significant antimicrobial activity against C. albicans and E. faecalis. Furthermore, it was observed by Garcia et al in 2009 that calcium hydroxide mixed with castor oil had better activity than calcium hydroxide mixed with propylene glycol against microorganisms commonly present in endodontic infections. [135]

4. Reprocessing endodontics

❖ Orange oil (Citrus sinensis), Eucalyptus oil (Eucalyptus globulus):

As endodontic desobturation is an important step in successful endodontic re-treatment, different methods are used to remove the obturation material, which are generally classified as thermal, mechanical, chemical or a combination of all three. As far as chemical desobturation is concerned, the solvents most commonly used in the past were chloroform, xylol, eucalyptol and turpentine oil. Xylol and chloroform are toxic for both patient and practitioner. Thus, it has been recommended in the literature to replace them with essential oils such as orange oil and eucalyptol, the main component of eucalyptus oil. [143] Studies have confirmed that products placed in the pulp chamber have access to periapical tissue and the circulatory system via the periodontal vascular system. Consequently, orange oil and eucalyptol have been proposed as more biocompatible products. [119]

Recent studies have indicated that orange oil, composed mainly of limonene, is as effective as xylene, chloroform and eucalyptol in softening gutta percha and dissolving endodontic sealants. [119,143]Moreover, orange oil has been shown to be effective in dissolving many endodontic sealants, such as those based on calcium hydroxide (Sealer 26), siliciumpolydimethylsiloxane(RoekoSeal) and zinc oxide-eugenol (Endofill and Intrafill) (Martos et al in 2011). [93]

For their part, Kulkarni et al in 2016 compared the ability of eucalyptus oil, orange oil and clove oil to dissolve resin-coated gutta-percha cones. The results showed that orange oil was the most effective of the solvents tested. [83]Orange oil is readily available, inexpensive, pleasant smelling and has antibacterial activity. In fact, an in vivo study carried out by Mohsen et al in 2022 showed that orange oil and eucalyptus oil have the following properties antibacterial against E.faecalis biofilm comparable to synthetic solvents (chloroform and xylene) during endodontic reprocessing. [22]

The dissolving action of lemon, unlike orange oil, has been little studied in the literature. The ability of grapefruit, mandarin, lime and lemon oils as solvents to soften gutta-percha in endodontic reprocessing procedures was investigated and compared with chloroform. The results revealed that chloroform was significantly the best solvent for softening gutta-percha, followed by grapefruit oil and mandarin oil, then lime oil and lemon oil. [75]

The solvent product of natural origin most recommended in the literature is orange oil while eucalyptol oil is not widely used because it does not effectively dissolve gutta percha at room temperature. [148]

5. Root canal fillings definitive

Ineffective root canal sealing can lead to the penetration of micro-organisms and reinfection, resulting in the failure of endodontic treatment. It is therefore important that the root canal sealing material has good antibacterial activity and provides a watertight seal.

❖ Copaiba oil :

Concerns about the toxicity and biocompatibility of resin-based sealants have prompted researchers to develop plant-based sealants to minimise the toxicity that can impair periapical healing. In this context, Reiznautt et al in 2020 conducted a study to evaluate the physicochemical properties, antimicrobial activity and cytocompatibility of resin-based endodontic sealants containing essential oils of butia capitata or copaiba. [120]

The commercial material used in this study was a methacrylate-based resin: RealSeal™

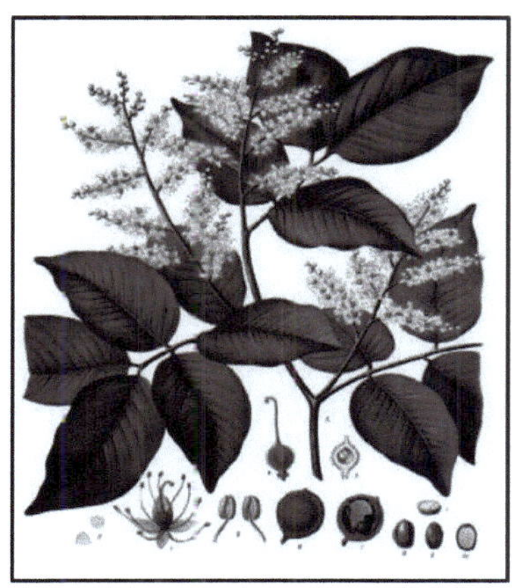

Figure 54: Copaifera officinalis [181].

Copaiba is a natural extract obtained from the trunk of the copaifera tree **(Figure 54).** The essential oil of the fruit of the Butia capitata tree has an antimicrobial effect attributed to the presence of long- and medium-chain fatty acids in its composition. [120] In the present study, Reiznautt et al found that the sealants tested had satisfactory cytocompatibility, antimicrobial effects and adequate physicochemical properties. These natural oil-containing materials caused less fibroblast cell death compared to RealSeal™. Thus, these sealants could be a promising alternative in endodontic practice. [120] In a previous study by Garrido et al in 2014, researchers developed a new Biosealer [BS] endodontic sealant composed of powder and liquid. The powder is composed of zinc oxide, calcium hydroxide, bismuth subcarbonate and sodium tetraborate and the liquid is a Copaiba oil-resin. [53]Copaiba oil has anti-inflammatory, analgesic, reparative, anti-nociceptive, anti-tumour and antimicrobial properties. In vitro results showed that the experimental Copaiba oil-resin sealant was not cytotoxic t o osteoblast-type cells. Nevertheless, more toxicity tests need to be performed in vivo before recommending this product for clinical application. [53]

❖ **Bixa orellana, Mentha piperita and Tagetes minuta :**

Another study, carried out by dos Santos et al in 2021, evaluated the antimicrobial activity and physical properties of experimental resin-based endodontic sealants with the incorporation of plant extracts obtained from the species **Bixa orellana (Roucouyer),** **Mentha piperita (Peppermint)** and **Tagetes minuta (Tagetes)** at mass concentrations of 0.5% by weight **(Figure 55,56,57).** A commercial RealSeal reference was used. [46]

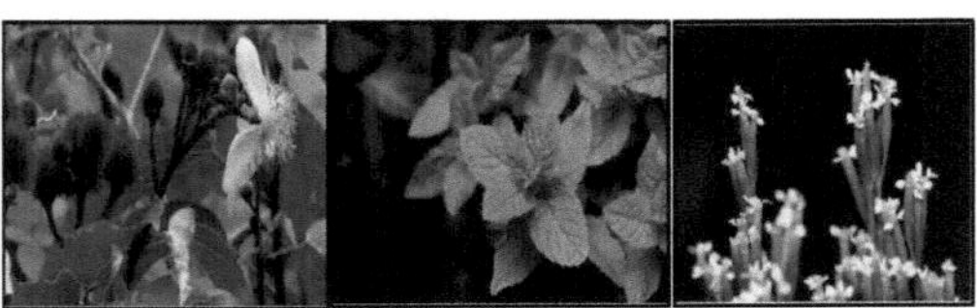

Figure 55: Roucouyer

(Bixa orellana) [162]

Figure 56: Peppermint (Mentha piperita) [160].

Figure 57: Tagetes (Tages minuta) [163].

The authors found that the addition of the plant extracts did not affect the physical properties of RealSeal. In addition, all the extracts showed an antibacterial effect against E. faecalis. However, for Streptococcus mutans, only the Tages minuta and Bixa orellana groups showed antibacterial activity after 24 h of contact.Bixa orellana's antibacterial activity is attributed to the presence of alkaloids and flavonoids and its ability to rupture bacterial membranes. It has also been shown to be safe and non-cytotoxic, even at high doses. In the case of Mentha Piperita, studies have demonstrated the inhibition of micro-organisms such as Escherichia coli, Staphylococcus aureus and C. albicans, even at low concentrations. The antimicrobial activities of Mentha Piperita and Tagetes minuta have been attributed to high levels of monoterpenes, exhibiting antimicrobial activity against both Gram (+) and Gram (-) bacteria[46].In the light of these results, dos Santos et al concluded that these experimental sealants show promise as new plant-based sealants. Nevertheless, further studies are needed. [46]

❖ Uncaria tomentosa (Cat's claw) :

Uncaria tomentosa (UT), also known as "cat's claw", is a plant of Amazonian origin belonging to the Rubiaceae family.It is known for its antioxidant, antimicrobial, antineoplastic, immunomodulatory, antiretroviral and anti-inflammatory properties. [44] In dentistry, this substance has shown promising results in the treatment of oral candidiasis, an antibacterial activity that has been shown to reduce the risk of infection. effective against human oral pathogens such as Enterococcus faecalis, Staphylococcus aureus and Candida albicans. [68]It has also been studied in gel form during the cleaning and shaping stage, or as a complement to the sealing cement during root canal obturation. Herrera et al in 2016 noted a similar reduction in bacterial load for 2% CHX, 2% UT gel and 2% sodium hypochlorite on E. Faecalis contaminated dentin. [67] In addition, the authors observed that both UT gel and CHX retained their antibacterial properties for up to 7 days after application. This property is known as substantivity. [67] Brazilian researchers have evaluated the cytotoxicity, antimicrobial and physicochemical properties of root canal sealants after incorporating 2% and 5% respectively of Uncaria tomentosa (UT).Unmodified AH Plus (Dentsply, DeTrey, Germany) and MTA Fillapex (Angelus, Londrina, Brazil) were used as controls. The results of this study showed that incorporation of Uncaria tomentosa decreased the cytotoxicity and increased the antimicrobial action of root canal sealants, without compromising their original physicochemical properties. [38]

Further studies are needed to determine whether the current results for AH Plus and MTA Fillapex are reproducible for other types of endodontic sealants. [38]

6. Post-traumatic dental avulsion

The prognosis of a reimplanted tooth depends on the extra-alveolar time and the storage medium. However, the capacity of the storage medium to preserve The vitality of periodontal ligament (PDL) cells attached to the root surface proved to be a key factor. Various storage media such as t a p water, saliva, saline, milk, culture media (Viaspan and Hank's balanced salt solution (HBSS)) have been described in the literature. However, these media have shown certain limitations. [59]In the search for new, safer and biocompatible storage media, several authors have studied plant-based products as storage media for avulsed teeth.

❖ Coconut water :

In 2008, Gopikrishna et al carried out a study evaluating the potential of a new storage medium, coconut water, for maintaining the viability of periodontal ligament (PDL) cells in simulated avulsed teeth. [59]Coconut water (Cocos nucifera L.) is a natural hypotonic solution that is biologically pure and sterile.The experimental teeth were kept dry for 30 minutes and then immersed in 1 of 3 media: coconut water (CW), Hank's balanced salt solution (HBSS) and milk; 30 minutes represents a typical clinical scenario during which the avulsed tooth can remain dry before being placed in a storage medium. The teeth were then treated with Dispase grade II and Collagenase for 30 minutes. Viable PDL cells were then counted using a haemocytometer. Coconut water was shown to maintain significantly more viable PDL cells than HBSS or milk. The result of this study is attributed to the composition of coconut water rich in proteins, amino acids, vitamins and minerals. [59]As the osmolarity of the transport medium is an important factor in maintaining the vitality of PDL cells, it has been reported that the growth of can occur in a range of 230 to 400 mOsm/l and a pH of (6.6 to 7.8). In the present study, the osmolarity of HBSS, milk and coconut water were found to be 295 mOsm/L, 232 mOsm/L and 372 mOsm/L respectively. [59] Similarly, Souza et al in 2016 observed that natural coconut water was significantly better at maintaining cell viability compared to Hank's balanced salt solution industrialised coconut water and milk. [139]

❖ Propolis :

Buttke & Trope in 2003 reported that the success of reimplantation can be increased by maintaining the avulsed teeth in a medium containing one or more antioxidants. Various authors have shown that propolis has antioxidant properties (Al-Shaher et al. 2004, Martin & Pileggi 2004).Propolis also contains iron and zinc, which are important for collagen synthesis and can increase the healing effect of epithelial tissue.According to a study by Martin et al in 2004, propolis was shown to maintain more viable periodontal ligament cells than milk, HBSS and saline. [92]Similarly, comparing a propolis solution to HBSS and milk, Ozan et al in 2007 found propolis to be a more effective storage medium than the other groups. The viability of PDL cells w a s assessed by trypan blue staining which is considered to be one of the most accurate methods of detecting remaining live cells. [106] Mahal et al in 2012 observed that there was no significant difference between HBSS, egg white and propolis in the maintenance of cell viability. In fact, egg white is a good preservation medium due to its high protein, vitamin and water content and lack of bacterial contamination. [85]

On the other hand, Gjertsen et al in 2011 conducted an in vitro study to assess not only the effect of propolis on the viability of periodontal ligament fibroblasts but also their proliferation. They observed that propolis decreased apoptosis and also increased metabolic activity and proliferation of PDL cells. [58] Propolis has shown promising results as a medium for preserving teeth avulsed after trauma. However, further studies are needed to determine a standard formula for therapeutic use.

❖ **Aloe vera :**

According to an in vitro study which evaluated the antioxidant activity of aloe vera used to preserve the vitality of the periodontal ligament cells of an expelled immature permanent tooth, the results showed that aloe vera has an antioxidant effect and that extracts of aloe vera gel at concentrations of 5 to 20% were able to preserve up to 95% of the vitality of the periodontal ligament cells for 24 hours and up to 65% for 72 hours at a concentration of 50%. [69] Furthermore, the ability of Aloe Vera extract at 10%,30% and 50% to maintain PDL cell viability was confirmed by Badakhsh et al in 2014. [28] Although these in vitro studies revealed the efficacy of Aloe vera extract in maintaining viable PDL cells, further research is essential to determine its ability to reduce or prevent complications that may arise after reimplantation, such as root resorptions.

❖ **Green tea :**

Green tea has been selected as a medium for the consevation of avulsed teeth because of its particular anti-inflammatory, anti-microbial and antioxidant properties. It also contains elements essential for cell growth such as calcium, magnesium, selenium, zinc, iron and fluoride, as well as certain carbohydrates such as glucose, fructose, sucrose and vitamins B, C and E [72].Green tea extract was found to be as effective as HBSS in maintaining PDL cell vitality and more effective than milk. [72]

On their part, Bharath et al in 2015 compared the efficacy of four preservation media (Hank's balanced salt solution, Ringer's lactate solution, tender coconut water and green tea extract) in maintaining the viability of human periodontal cells at different time intervals 15,30, 60 and 90 min. It was shown that there was no difference in cell viability between the four media up to a period of 60 min, whereas green tea extract showed lower cell viability after 90 min. [34]

Natural products have shown good results in terms of preserving the vitality of PDL cells in expelled teeth. Nevertheless, considering other criteria in the choice of the best preservation medium for avulsed teeth such as availability and cost-effectiveness, the most recommended medium in the literature was milk, followed by HBSS. [7]

7. Regeneration endodontics

❖ **Morinda citrifolia :**

In the context of endodontic regeneration, where the aim is to re-establish an environment favourable to cell recruitment, migration and proliferation, it is recommended that irrigation solutions be used which provide optimum disinfection while allowing the survival of progenitor stem cells.Indeed, it has been reported in the literature that 5% NAOCL and 2%

CHX have a cytotoxic effect on stem cells (Martin et al, 2014 Widbiller et al, 2019) Therefore, it has been recommended to use a low concentration of 1.5% NaOCl in regeneration procedures (Martin et al., 2014 Trevino et al., 2011). However, controversy remains over the ability of low concentrations of NaOCl to completely eradicate infected biofilms (Ma et al, 2015 Tagelsir et al, 2016). [90,94]

So it's important to look for alternative antimicrobial products of natural origin. In this context, Al Moghazy et al in 2018 conducted a study that aimed to compare the effect of different irrigation solutions, including Morinda citrifolia (MC) as a natural irrigant on the attachment of human dental pulp stem cells to the dentin walls of the root canal using scanning electron microscopy(SEM). The MC with EDTA group (17%) had a statistically significant higher mean cell count compared with MC alone, the NaOCL 5.25% group and the NaOCL 5.25% group combined with 17% EDTA. EDTA superficially demineralises the dentinal walls of the roots, allowing the release of growth factors immobilised in the matrix of dentin. These growth factors will promote neoangiogenesis and secondarily participate in the recruitment, proliferation, survival and differentiation of the stem cells involved in the regeneration process. At the end of this study, it was concluded that this combination (MC and EDTA) promotes adhesion and attachment of pulpal stem cells to the walls of the root canal hence the usefulness of using Morinda citrifolia as an irrigation solution in future regenerative endodontic practice. [14]

❖ Chrysine :

Chrysin (5,7-dihydroxyflavone) is a natural flavonoid that is considered an active ingredient in honey, passion fruit, Indian trumpet flower and European propolis. [16] Flavonoids are part of the family of bioactive polyphenols that exist in the plant kingdom. Chrysin has been shown to have antibacterial and anti-inflammatory activity and to induce osteogenic differentiation and mineralisation. The latter property is essential for dentinal wall thickening, root development and apical closure. Because of these interesting properties, a study was carried out to evaluate chrysin for its anti-oxidant, anti-inflammatory and mineralisation properties on dental pulp stem cells (DPSC). [16]

To overcome the limitations of chrysin, it was loaded onto polycaprolactone-gelatin scaffolds. Poly (ε-caprolactone) (PCL) is a biodegradable and biocompatible polymer with various applications in regenerative medicine and gelatin is a natural polymer, which induces DPSC colonisation and pulp tissue revascularisation. [16]   The results of the study showed that chrysin-loaded scaffolds have antibacterial activity against 4 bacterial strains (Acinetobacterbaumannii, Pseudomonasaeruginosa, Staphylococcus aureus and Enterococcus faecalis) involved in endodontic infection, in addition to anti-oxidant and anti-inflammatory activity. [16] ALP enzyme activity and the formation of mineralised stem cell nodules on the scaffolds were significantly increased compared with the chrysin-free control group.During dentinogenesis, undifferentiated dental pulp stem cells differentiate into odontoblasts, which synthesise type 1 collagen and alkaline phosphatase. These results indicated that chrysin can promote odontoblastic differentiation of dental pulp stem cells in addition to eliminating infection and inflammation making it a promising alternative for regeneration of the dentin-pulp complex. [16]

❖ **Propolis :**

According to a study by El-Tayeb et al in 2019 evaluating the antibacterial activity of propolis and its ability to promote endodontic regeneration of necrotic immature permanent teeth in dogs when used as a root canal plug after revascularisation, the results showed that there was no significant difference between the groups treated with triple antibiotic paste (TAP) and propolis paste in terms of antibacterial efficacy. [49]

Triple antibiotic paste containing minocycline, metronidazole and ciprofloxacin has the potential side-effects of discolouring teeth and also causes demineralisation of dentine, increasing the risk of fracture. In addition, in high concentrations, it has a on pulp stem cells, hindering the regeneration process. [94,143]

Therefore, propolis was used in the present study as an alternative intra-canal drug due to its anti-inflammatory, antibacterial and biocompatibility properties. [49]

After a disinfection period of 3 weeks, revascularisation was induced in all experimental teeth. The Propolis and MTA treated groups showed a similar response in terms of increased root length and dentin thickness, new hard tissue formation and vital tissue formation within the pulp canal. [49]

A study by Pagliarin et al in 2016 showed similar results. In fact, there were no statistically significant differences between the experimental groups in the formation of new mineralised tissue and further root development. However, the propolis group showed more vital tissue in the root canals (100%) than the TAP group (70%). The authors attributed this result to the fact that propolis paste has minimal toxicity and therefore induced cell proliferation. The new tissues formed inside the root canal showed characteristics similar to cementum, bone and periodontal ligament. [107]

The results of these studies have shown that propolis paste can be a substitute for triple antibiotic paste and MTA in the revascularisation procedure for immature permanent teeth, with the advantage of not causing dyschromia in the teeth. Similar studies in humans a r e therefore recommended. [49,107]

❖ **Curcumin :**

Sinjari et al in 2019 studied the direct contact of curcumin-loaded liposome nanocarriers with dental pulp stem cells in the presence of hydrophilic monomers (2-Hydroxyethyl Methacrylate) HEMA. [94] The results indicated that the latter are capable of blocking the secretion of inflammatory cytokines by inhibiting the NFkB/ERK/ pERK signalling cascade and stimulate the proliferation of stem cells, but are not involved in odontoblastic differentiation.In addition, Alipour et al in 2021 evaluated the ability of curcumin-loaded polycaprolactone(PCL)-Gelatin scaffold to reduce infection and inflammation in addition to inducing mineralisation during healing of the dentin-pulp complex. [15] The results showed that the PCL/Gelatin/Curcumin scaffold had antibacterial, antioxidant and anti-inflammatory effects by inhibiting tumour necrosis factor a and DCF of inflamed human dental pulp stem cells (hDPSCs). In addition, the curcumin-loaded material provided a suitable structure for stem cell attachment and proliferation. [15]

8. Bone regeneration in endodontic surgery

Endodontic surgery is generally indicated in cases of failed treatment or orthograde endodontic retreatment of teeth with apical lesions. [33]

As far as bone regeneration is concerned there are almost no studies directly evaluating the use of plants in apical surgery. However, studies have evaluated the application of natural products in bone regeneration.

❖ Propolis :

According to a study conducted by Yuanita et al in 2018 that aimed to investigate propolis as a potential natural intracanal drug for the prevention of bone resorption of induced chronic apical periodontitis in Wistar rats, the results showed that propolis increased the expression of osteoprotegerin(OPG) (a potential inhibitor of osteoclastogenesis) and decreased the number of osteoclasts. Indeed, OPG inhibits osteoclast differentiation by binding to RANK with high affinity, thus preventing RANKL from binding to its cognate receptor, RANK. [155]
Similarly, a previous study by Anhangari et al in 2013 demonstrated that caffeic acid phenethyl ester, a main component of propolis has the ability to inhibit osteoclast activity by suppressing nuclear factor kappa B which is activated in osteoclastogenesis. [33]
In addition, Zohery et al in 2018 compared the efficacy of Egyptian propolis with nanohydroxyapatite grafting on the regeneration of furcation defects in dogs. The results indicated a significant increase in inter-radicular bone height with high osteoblast activity for the collagen/propolis group compared to the collagen/nanohydroxyapatite group. [156]
Propolis through its antioxidant action and ability to potentiate cell proliferation and inhibit bone resorption has proven to be an osteoconductive and osteinductive material that can be used for the management of bone defects. [156]

❖ Acemannan :

Acemannan is an acetylated(1-4) polymannose extracted from Aloe vera gel. According to a study evaluating the acemannan sponge effect on proliferation, differentiation, extracellular matrix synthesis and the formation of primary bone marrow stromal cells in a rat model of dental extraction, in vivo results showed that acemannan-treated groups had higher bone mineral density and faster bone healing compared with acemannan-untreated controls. The authors concluded that acemannan could be a natural biomaterial with potential for bone regeneration. In addition, acemannan also accelerated the formation of new alveolar bone, cementum and periodontal ligament in canine class II furcation defects. [142]
Two randomised controlled trials with a 12-month observation period evaluated bone regeneration after acemannan sponge treatment following tooth extraction and apical surgery, respectively. [84,149] The results of the radiographic evaluations showed that the use of acemannan sponge significantly improved the rate of bone healing without any side effects. At 3-month follow-up, the reduction in the volume of bone defects in the acemannan groups was greater than in the control group (without acemannan sponge), and similar results were observed at 6 and 12 months. Acemannan has been shown to be an osteoinductive biomaterial that can be safely used in apical surgery. However, a longer observation period of up to 5 years after apical surgery is recommended. Indeed, it would clearly confirm the efficacy and safety of using acemannan sponge. [84]

Table 1: Areas of use of plants in endodontics and examples of plants that can be used for each indication, according to the literature.

Clinical indication	Examples of plants
Preserving pulp vitality	propolis acemannan Nigella oil (Nigella sativa) Turmeric (Curcuma Longa) Thyme (Thymus vulgaris) Allium Sativum (Garlic) oil Aloe Vera gel
Root canal irrigation	Morinda Citrifolia Propolis Azadirachta Indica (Neem) Triphala Green tea (Camellia Sinensis) Acacia Nilotica Garlic (Allium Sativum) Grape seed extract (Vitis Vinifera) Turmeric (Curcuma Longa) Clove (Syzygium aromaticum) Cinnamon (Cinnamomum zeylanicum) Tea tree oil (Melaleuca alternifolia) Meswak (Salvadora Persica) German chamomile (Matricaria recutita) Passion fruit (Passiflora edulis) Guava (Psidium Guajava) FéruleGommeus(FérulaGummosa) Carvacrol Myrtle (Myrtus communis) Nutmeg (Myristica fragrans) Lemon solution Jieeryin's solution
Intracanal medication	Casearia sylvestris Swartz Papain Morinda citrifolia Tulsi (Ocimum Sanctum or Ocimum tenuiflorum) Propolis Azadirachta Indica (Neem) Garlic (Allium sativum) Great burdock (Arctium lappa) Aloe vera gel Licorice (Glycyrrhiza glabra) Cumin (Cuminum cyminum) Castor oil (Ricinus communis) Uncaria tomentosa (Cat's claw)
Endodontic treatment	Orange oil (Citrus sinensis) Eucalyptus oil (Eucalyptus globulus) Lemon oil

Sealing in definitive root canal obturation (incorporation of medicinal plants in root canal sealing cements)	Butia capitata and Copaiba essential oils Bixa orellana, Mentha piperita and Tagetes minuta Uncaria tomentosa (Cat's claw)
Preservation media for teeth avulsed following trauma	Coconut water Propolis Green tea Aloe vera
Endodontic regeneration	Morinda citrifolia Chrysine Propolis Curcumin
Bone regeneration	Acemannan Propolis

UNDESIRABLE EFFECTS AND DRUG INTERACTIONS

The literature has discussed a variety of herbs with potential for use as innovative alternatives in endodontics, reporting adverse reactions and drug interactions between herbal products and conventional medicines. However, it is notable that few adverse reactions have been reported in the field of herbal dentistry.

Despite the various therapeutic effects reported in endodontics, a study by Ahangari et al. in 2013 highlighted that the application of 30% propolis as an intracanal medication resulted in tooth dyschromia. [9]

In addition, this staining is irreversible and was not removed despite the removal of the product from the root canal (Ahangari et al. 2021). [11]

In addition, eugenol, commonly used in dentistry for its analgesic and antibacterial properties, has been shown to have negative effects on the soft tissues of the oral cavity. Eugenol has an allergenic effect and can induce a localised delayed hypersensitivity reaction. It is also generally cytotoxic in high concentrations and has a harmful effect on fibroblasts and osteoblast-like cells. In addition, the literature reports a case of a particularly sensitive patient who developed anaphylactic shock following pulpotomy with zinc oxide eugenol. [124]

Similarly, tea tree oil, castor oil and Allium sativum extract can cause allergic contact dermatitis (Khanna et al, 2000; Fritz et al, 2001). Indeed, turpentine (limonene, alpha-pinene, phellandrene) an essential component of tea tree oil is potentially allergenic. [36] Other reported side effects of castor oil include nausea, vomiting and colic, as well as a laxative effect. On the other hand, it has been reported that washing the eyes with chamomile (Matricaria chamomilla) can induce allergic conjunctivitis (Subiza et al, 1990). [37]

Topical aloe vera gel can cause allergic contact dermatitis and increase the absorption of local corticoids.

Orally, Aloe vera has laxative properties and may be associated with abdominal pain. It also interacts with oral antidiabetics and insulin, potentiating their effects, as well as diuretics or laxatives such as sevoflurane or digoxin. [141]Chamomile in combination with aspirin or warfarin increases the risk of bleeding. When combined with benzodiazepines, it causes increased sedation. [37,82]

Garlic taken orally can cause irritation of the intestines, ulceration of the mouth and halitosis. It interacts with anticoagulants, increasing the risk of bleeding, and with hypoglycaemic and hypotensive drugs, amplifying their effects. [99,82] Orange oil causes gastrointestinal irritation when taken orally, while green tea reduces the bioavailability of anti-cancer drugs. [82]In addition, it has been reported in the literature that green tea reduces the anticoagulant effect of warfarin. This may be due to its high vitaminK. [82] The scientific literature has explored various potential applications of plants in endodontics. However, there is still a lack of clinical studies on the actual effectiveness of these natural products in endodontics, their biocompatibility, their possible adverse effects and their possible interactions with other drugs.

CONCLUSION

Medicinal plants have been extensively studied in the treatment of a number of oral and dental diseases, particularly in endodontics.The results of the in vitro and in vivo literature have shown a number of clinical applications, in particular as pulp capping or pulpotomy agents, root canal irrigants, intracanal drugs, conservation media for permanent teeth avulsed following trauma, gutta percha solvents during endodontic re-treatment, sealing materials during root canal obturation and also as materials promoting bone and endodontic regeneration.Thanks to their antibacterial activity, natural products have shown the ability to eradicate biofilms of bacteria involved in endodontic infection, in particular E.faecalis, and have shown anti-inflammatory, antioxidant and regenerative activity comparable to certain conventional products.Plant-based products offer a number of advantages, including safety, availability, increased shelf life, cost-effectiveness and lack of bacterial resistance. The diversity of methodological approaches in published in vitro and in vivo studies, such as the method of preparation of plant extracts, extract concentrations, time of harvest and botanical origin, as well as the different methods of data analysis, make it impossible to reach specific recommendations for the use of plant-based products in clinical practice. In addition, data in the literature on possible side effects is limited. This justifies the need for additional studies with a high level of scientific evidence, using up-to-date protocols and techniques to assess biocompatibility, efficacy, the risk of tooth discolouration with long-term use and possible interactions with other products.Numerous studies have highlighted the beneficial properties of phytotherapy compared with conventional products. However, clinical data is scarce, which is why it is so important to increase research efforts and funding for clinical trials.

REFERENCES

1. **Abbasi M, Norouzifard A, Sharifi M.**
In Vitro Antifungal Efficacy of Different Intracanal Irrigants against Candida Albicans.
J Iran Dent Assoc 2015;27(1):15-8.

2. **Abbaszadegan A, Gholami A, Ghahramani Y et al.** Antimicrobial and Cytotoxic Activity of Cuminum Cyminum as an Intracanal Medicament Compared to Chlorhexidine Gel.
Iran Endod J 2016;11(1):44-50.

3. **Abbaszadegan A, Gholami A, Mirhadi H, Saliminasab M, Kazemi A, Moein MR.**
Antimicrobial and cytotoxic activity of Ferula gummosa plant essential oil compared to NaOCl and CHX: a preliminary in vitro study.
Restor Dent Endod 2015;40(1):50-7.

4. **Abbaszadegan A, Sahebi S, Gholami A et al.**
Time-dependent antibacterial effects of Aloe vera and Zataria multiflora plant essential oils compared to calcium hydroxide in teeth infected with Enterococcus faecalis.
J Investig Clin Dent 2016;7(1):93-101.

5. **Abdeltawab SS, Abu Haimed TS, Bahammam HA, Arab WT, Abou Neel EA, Bahammam LA.**
Biocompatibility and Antibacterial Action of Salvadora persica Extract as Intracanal Medication (In Vitro and Ex Vivo Experiment).
Materials 2022;15(4):1-19.

6. **Adel M, Pourrousta P, Sharifi M, Javadi A, Falah-Abed P, Rahmani N.**
Antimicrobial Effect of Carvacrol and Calcium Hydroxide against
Enterococcus Faecalis in Different Layers of Dentin and Different Time Intervals.
J Mazandaran Univ Med Sci 2016;26:35-43.

7. **Adnan S, Lone MM, Khan FR, Hussain SM, Nagi SE.**
Which is the most recommended medium for the storage and transport of avulsed teeth? A systematic review.
Dent Traumatol 2018;34(2):59-70.

8. **Agrawal V, Kapoor S, Agrawal I.**
Critical Review on Eliminating Endodontic Dental Infections Using
Herbal Products.
J Diet Suppl 2017;14(2):229-40.

9. **Ahangari Z, Ghassemi A, Shamszadeh S, Naseri M.**
The Effects of Propolis on Discoloration of Teeth.
J Dent School 2013; 31(1):33-41

10. **Ahangari Z, Mashhadiabbas F, Feli M, Jafari Z, Zadsirjan S.** Evaluation of Pulp Tissue Following Direct Pulp Capping with Propolis versus Calcium Hydroxide: A Clinical Trial.
J Dent School 2020;38(4):134-8.

11. **Ahangari Z, Naseri M, Banihashem S, Namjou S, Eftekhar L.** Effect of Propolis Application in Root Canal Therapy for Decontamination; Reversible or Irreversible Coronal Discoloration? J Dent Materials Tech 2021;10:102-7.

12. **Aini FN, Adiningrat A.**
Challenge in Propolis Biocompatibility as a Potential Medicament in Dental Medicine: A Literature Review.
Adv Health Sci Res 2020;33 :237-47.

13. **Akhtar J, Siddique KM, Bi S, Mujeeb M.**
A review on phytochemical and pharmacological investigations of miswak (Salvadora persica Linn).
J Pharm Bioallied Sci 2011;3(1):113-7.

14. **Al Moghazy HH, El Shafei JM, Abulezz EH, El Baz AA.**
The Effect of Morinda citrifolia in Combination with Chelating Agent EDTA on Isolated and Differentiated Human Dental Pulp Stem Cells Attachment to Root Canal Dentine Walls.
Acta Sci Dent Sci 2018;2:6-11.

15. **Alipour M, Fadakar S, Aghazadeh M et al.**
Synthesis, characterization, and evaluation of curcumin-loaded endodontic reparative material.
J Biochem Mol Toxicol 2021;35(9):1-9.

16. **Alipour M, Pouya B, Aghazadeh Z et al.**
The Antimicrobial, Antioxidative, and Anti-Inflammatory Effects of Polycaprolactone/Gelatin Scaffolds Containing Chrysin for
Regenerative Endodontic Purposes.
Stem Cells Int. 2021;2021:1-11.

17. **Aljarbou F, Niazy AA, Lambarte RN et al.**
Efficacy of Salvadora persica root extract as an endodontic irrigant-An in-vitro evaluation. J Herbal Med 2022;34.

18. **Almadi EM, Almohaimede AA.** Natural products in endodontics. Saudi Med J 2018;39(2):124-30.

19. **Al-Qathami H, Al-Madi E.**
Comparison of sodium hypochlorite, propolis and saline as root canal irrigants: A pilot study. Saudi Dent J 2003;15:1-5.

20. **Al-Sabawi NA, Al Sheikh Abdal A, Taha MY.**
The antimicrobial activity of Salvadora persica solution (miswak- siwak) as root canal irrigant (a comparative study).
Univ Sharjah J Pure Appl Sci 2007;4(3):69-91.

21. **Ambareen Z, Chinappa A.**
Go Green- Keep the Root Canal Clean!!!
Int J Dent Sci Res 2014;2(6B):21-5.

22. **Aminsobhani M, Razmi H, Hamidzadeh F, Rezaei Avval A.** Evaluation of the Antibacterial Effect of Xylene, Chloroform, Eucalyptol, and Orange Oil on Enterococcus

faecalis in Nonsurgical Root Canal Retreatment: An Ex Vivo Study.
Biomed Res Int 2022;2022:1-9.

23. Anusuya V, Jena AK, Sharan J.

Grape Seed Extracts in Dental Therapy. In: Chauhan DN, Singh PR,
Shah K, Chauhan NS, eds. Natural Oral Care in Dental Therapy. 1st ed.
Hoboken, New Jersey, USA: John Wiley & Sons, 2020:229-58.

24. Arslan S, Ozbilge H, Kaya EG, Er O.

In vitro antimicrobial activity of propolis, BioPure MTAD, sodium
hypochlorite, and chlorhexidine on Enterococcus faecalis and Candida albicans.
Saudi Med J 2011;32(5):479-83.

25. Awawdeh L, Al-Beitawi M, Hammad M.

Effectiveness of propolis and calcium hydroxide as a short-term intracanal medicament
against Enterococcus faecalis: a laboratory study.
Aust Endod J 2009;35(2):52-8.

26. Awawdeh L, Jamleh A, Al Beitawi M.

The Antifungal Effect of Propolis Endodontic Irrigant with Three Other
Irrigation Solutions in Presence and Absence of Smear Layer: An In Vitro Study.
Iran Endod J 2018;13(2):234-9.

27. Ayoub N, Badr N, Alghamdi S et al.

The Effectiveness of Salavadora Persica (Siwak) Petroleum Ether Extract As An Intracanal
Medicament Used in Endodontic Therapy: An In Vitro Study.
Res Square 2021 [Preprint]. DOI: https://doi.org/10.21203/rs.3.rs- 219563/v1

28. Badakhsh S, Eskandarian T, Esmaeilpour T.

The use of aloe vera extract as a novel storage media for the avulsed tooth
Iran J Med Sci 2014;39(4):327-32.

29. Baranwal R, Duggi V, Avinash A, Dubey A, Pagaria S, Munot H.

Propolis: A Smart Supplement for an Intracanal Medicament.

Int J Clin Pediatr Dent 2017;10(4):324-9.

30. Bardají DK, Reis EB, Medeiros TC, Lucarini R, Crotti AE, Martins CH.
Antibacterial activity of commercially available plant-derived essential oils against oral
pathogenic bacteria.
Nat Product Res 2016;30(10):1178-81.

**31. Bazvand L, Aminozarbian MG, Farhad A, Noormohammadi H, Hasheminia SM,
Mobasherizadeh S.**
Antibacterial effect of triantibiotic mixture, chlorhexidine gel, and two natural materials
Propolis and Aloe vera against Enterococcus faecalis: An ex vivo study.
Dent Res J 2014;11(4):469-74.

32. Bedier Messrs.

Comparative Evaluation of the Antibacterial Activity of Cinnamon
zylanicum (True Cinnamon) and Azadirachta indica (Neem) Herbal Extracts Versus Calcium
Hydroxide Intracanal Medication against Enterococcus faecalis in Single Rooted Premolars

Teeth: A
Randomized In Vitro Study.
Acta Sci Dent Sci 2020;11:1-9.

33. **Benetti F, Bueno CR.**
Phytotherapy in endodontics. In: Bueno CR, ed. Contemporary Use of Plant Extracts in Dentistry: Scientific Evidence for Phytotherapy and Ethnopharmacology.
New York: Nova Science Pub Inc; 2020: 1-39.

34. **Bharath MJ, Sahadev CK, Ramachandra PK, Rudranaik S, George J, Thomas A.**
Comparative evaluation of four transport media for maintaining cell viability in transportation of an avulsed tooth - An in vitro study.
J Int Soc Prev Community Dent 2015;5(1):69-73.

35. **Bhardwaj A, Ballal S, Velmurugan N.**
Comparative evaluation of the antimicrobial activity of natural extracts of Morinda citrifolia, papain and aloe vera (all in gel
formulation), 2% chlorhexidine gel and calcium hydroxide, against Enterococcus faecalis: An in vitro study.
J Conserv Dent 2012;15(3):293-7.

36. **Bhargava KY, Aggarwal S, Kumar T, Bhargava S.**
Comparative evaluation of the efficacy of three anti-oxidants vs NaOCl and EDTA: Used for root canal irrigation in smear layer removal-SEM study.
Int J Pharm Sci 2015;7:366-71.

37. **Buggapati L.**
Herbs in dentistry.
Int J Pharm Sci Invent 2016;5(6):7-12.

38. **Caldas NL, Prado MC, Carvalho NK, Senna PM, Silva EJ.** Cytotoxicity, and antimicrobial and physicochemical properties of sealers incorporated with Uncaria tomentosa.
Braz Oral Res 2021;35:1-9.

39. **Carbajal Mejía JB.**
Antimicrobial effects of calcium hydroxide, chlorhexidine, and propolis on Enterococcus faecalis and Candida albicans.
J Investig Clin Dent 2014;5(3):194-200.

40. **Cecchin D, Soares Giaretta V, Granella Cadorin B, Albino Souza M, Vidal CMP, Paula Farina A.**
Effect of synthetic and natural-derived novel endodontic irrigant solutions on mechanical properties of human dentin.
J Mater Sci Mater Med 2017;28(9):1-6.

41. **Chandrappa PM, Dupper A, Tripathi P, Arroju R, Sharma P, Sulochana K.**
Antimicrobial activity of herbal medicines (tulsi extract, neem extract) and chlorhexidine against Enterococcus faecalis in Endodontics: An in vitro study.
J Int Soc Prev Community Dent 2015;5:S89-92.

42. **Clément RP.**
The roots of phytotherapy: between tradition and modernity (Part 1).
Phytotherapie 2005;3(4):171-5.

43. **Dadresanfar B, Vatanpour M, Farahmand M, Taheri S, Mahaseni Aghdam HR.**
Ex Vivo Comparative Study of the Effect of Different Concentrations of Green Tea Extract and Two Common Irrigants on Root Canals Infected with Enterococcus faecalis.
J Res Dent Maxillofac Sci 2019;4(2):32-6.

44. **Dioguardi M, Spirito F, Sovereto D, Ballini A, Alovisi M, Lo Muzio L.**
Application of the Extracts of Uncaria tomentosa in Endodontics and Oral Medicine: Scoping Review.
J Clin Med 2022;11(17):1-11.

45. **Divia AR, Nair MG, Varughese JM, Kurien S.**
A comparative evaluation of Morinda citrifolia, green tea polyphenols, and Triphala with 5% sodium hypochlorite as an endodontic irrigant against Enterococcus faecalis: An in vitro study.
Dent Res J 2018;15(2):117-22.

46. **Dos Santos DC, da Silva Barboza A, Schneider LR et al.** Antimicrobial and physical properties of experimental endodontic sealers containing vegetable extracts.
Sci Rep 2021;11(1):1-10.

47. **Dubey S.**
Comparative antimicrobial efficacy of herbal alternatives (Emblica officinalis, Psidium guajava), MTAD, and 2.5% sodium hypochlorite against Enterococcus faecalis: An in vitro study.
J Oral Biol Craniofac Res 2016;6(1):45-8.

48. **Ege B, Ege M..**
Therapeutic applications of phytopharmaceuticals in dentistry. In: Chauhan DN, Shah K, eds. Phytopharmaceuticals: Potential Therapeutic Applications.
Hoboken, New Jersey: John Wiley & Sons ; 2021 :191-222.

49. **El-Tayeb MM, Abu-Seida AM, El Ashry SH, El-Hady SA.** Evaluation of antibacterial activity of propolis on regenerative potential of necrotic immature permanent teeth in dogs.
BMC Oral Health 2019;19(1):1-12.

50. **Farhad Mollashahi N, Bokaeian M, Farhad Mollashahi L, Afrougheh A.**
Antifungal Efficacy of Green Tea Extract against Candida Albicans Biofilm on Tooth Substrate.
J Dent 2015;12(8):592-8.

51. **Fiallos NM, Cecchin D, de Lima CO, Hirata R Jr, Silva EJN, Sassone LM.**
Antimicrobial efficacy of grape seed extract against Enterococcus faecalis biofilm: A Confocal Laser Scanning Microscopy analysis.
Aust Endod J 2020;46(2):191-6.

52. **Garg P, Tyagi SP, Sinha DJ, Singh UP, Malik V, Maccune ER.** Comparison of antimicrobial efficacy of propolis, Morinda citrifolia, Azadirachta indica, triphala, green tea polyphenols and 5.25% sodium hypochlorite against Enterococcus fecalis biofilm.

Saudi Endod J 2014;4(3):122-7.

53. **Garrido AD, de Cara SP, Marques MM, Sponchiado EC, Garcia Lda F, de Sousa-Neto MD.**
Cytotoxicity evaluation of a copaiba oil-based root canal sealer compared to three commonly used sealers in endodontics.
Dent Res J 2015;12(2):121-6.

54. **Gayathri K, G.S P, Sajeev R, Sanguida A.**
Antimicrobial efficacy of passion fruit extract against enterococcus faecalis - an in vitro study. Int J Sci Res 2020;9 :1-3.

55. **Ghasemi N, Behnezhad M, Asgharzadeh M, Zeinalzadeh E, Kafil HS.** Antibacterial properties of aloe vera on intracanal medicaments against Enterococcus faecalis biofilm at different stages of development.
Int J Dent2020; 2020:1-6.

56. **Ghasemi Y, Faridi P, Mehregan I, Mohagheghzadeh A** Ferula gummosa Fruits: An Aromatic Antimicrobial Agent. Chem Nat Comp 2005;41:311-4.

57. **Ghonmode WN, Balsaraf OD, Tambe VH, Saujanya KP, Patil AK, Kakde DD.**
Comparison of the antibacterial efficiency of neem leaf extracts, grape seed extracts and 3% sodium hypochlorite against E. feacalis - An in
vitro study.
J Int Oral Health 2013;5(6):61-6.

58. **Gjertsen AW, Stothz KA, Neiva KG, Pileggi R.**
Effect of propolis on proliferation and apoptosis of periodontal ligament fibroblasts.
Oral Surg Oral Med Oral Pathol Oral Radiol Endod 2011;112(6):843-8.

59. **Gopikrishna V, Thomas T, Kandaswamy D.**
A quantitative analysis of coconut water: a new storage media for avulsed teeth.
Oral Surg Oral Med Oral Pathol Oral Radiol Endod. 2008;105(2):e61-5.

60. **Gupta A, Duhan J, Sangwan P, Hans S, Goyal V.**
The effectiveness of three different plant extracts used as irrigant in removal of smear layer: A scanning electron microscopic study.
J Oral Health Community Dent 2015;9:16-22.

61. **Gupta A, Duhan J, Tewari S et al.**
Comparative evaluation of antimicrobial efficacy of Syzygium aromaticum, Ocimum sanctum and Cinnamomum zeylanicum plant extracts against Enterococcus faecalis: a preliminary study.
Int Endod J 2013;46(8):775-83.

62. **Gupta D, Kamat S, Hugar S, Nanjannawar G, Kulkarni R.**
A comparative evaluation of the antibacterial efficacy of Thymus vulgaris, Salvadora persica, Acacia nilotica, Calendula arvensis, and 5% sodium hypochlorite against Enterococcus faecalis: An in-vitro study.
J Conserv Dent. 2020;23(1):97-101.

63. **Gupta-Wadhwa A, Wadhwa J, Duhan J.**
Comparative evaluation of antimicrobial efficacy of three herbal irrigants in reducing intracanal E. faecalis populations: An in vitro study.
J Clin Exp Dent 2016;8(3):e230-5.

64. **Hajlaoui H, Mighri H, Noumi E et al.**
Chemical composition and biological activities of Tunisian Cuminum cyminum L. essential oil: a high effectiveness against Vibrio spp. strains.
Food Chem Toxicol 2010;48(8-9):2186-92.

65. **Hashem SN, Fawzy MI, Mostafa MH.**
Comparative Study of Some Natural Materials Versus Traditional Medicaments used for Pulp Treatment of Primary Teeth.
Al-Azhar Dent J . 2019;6(1):25-30.

66. **Hegde M, Shetty S, Patil M, Patil A.**
An in vitro evaluation of antimicrobial activity of aqueous Curcuma longa ex- tract against endodontic pathogens.
Int J Res Phytochem Pharmacol 2012;2:1-6.

67. **Herrera DR, Durand-Ramirez JE, Falcão A, Silva EJ, Santos EB, Gomes BP.**
Antimicrobial activity and substantivity of Uncaria tomentosa in infected root canal dentin.
Braz Oral Res 2016;30(1):e61.

68. **Herrera DR, Tay LY, Rezende EC, Kozlowski Jr VA, Santos EB.** In vitro antimicrobial activity of phytotherapic Uncaria tomentosa against endodontic pathogens.
J Oral Sci 2010;52:473-6.

69. **Hortense MM, Julien NJ, Emmanuel NN, Kattie AL.**
Antioxidant Activity of Aloe Schureenfurthii and Maintenance of Vitality of Periodontal Cells of an Expelled Immature Permanent Tooth. Health Sciences Dis 2021;22 :71-6.

70. **Hotwani K, Baliga S, Sharma K.**
Phytodentistry: use of medicinal plants.
J Complement Integr Med 2014;11(4):233-51.

71. **Hugar SM, Kukreja P, Hugar SS, Gokhale N, Assudani H.** Comparative Evaluation of Clinical and Radiographic Success of Formocresol, Propolis, Turmeric Gel, and Calcium Hydroxide on Pulpotomized Primary Molars: A Preliminary Study.
Int J Clin Pediatr Dent 2017;10(1):18-23.

72. **Hwang JY, Choi SC, Park JH, Kang SW.**
The use of green tea extract as a storage medium for the avulsed tooth.
J Endod 2011;37(7):962-7.

73. **Jain G.**
Comparative Evaluation of Antimicrobial efficacy of Guava Leaf Extract, Asafetida Extract and 2.5% Sodium Hypochlorite used as Endodontic Irrigant: An In-vitro study.
Group 2020;1 :117-25.

74. **Jain PA, Tejaswi S, Parinitha M, Shetty S, Ambikathanaya U.** Comparative evaluation of antibacterial activity of Punica granatum, Acacia nilotica and Emblica officinalis against Enterococcus faecalis and their smear layer removal ability when used as endodontic irrigants: An in-vitro study.
Int J Res Rev. 2019;6(8):184-94.

75. **Jantarat J, Malhotra W, Sutimuntanakul S.**
Efficacy of grapefruit, tangerine, lime, and lemon oils as solvents for softening gutta-percha in root canal retreatment procedures.
J Investig Clin Dent 2013;4(1):60-3.

76. **Jayahari NK, Niranjan NT, Kanaparthy A.**
The efficacy of passion fruit juice as an endodontic irrigant compared with sodium hypochlorite solution: an in vitro study.
J Investig Clin Dent 2014;5(2):154-60.

77. **Jha S, Goel N, Dash BP, Sarangal H, Garg I, Namdev R.**
An Update on Newer Pulpotomy Agents in Primary Teeth: A Literature Review.
J Pharm Bioallied Sci 2021;13:57-61.

78. **Jorite S.**
Phytotherapy, a discipline between past and future: from herbalism to natural pharmacies [Thesis].
Bordeaux: U.F.R des Sciences pharmaceutiques, 2015.

79. **Joy Sinha D, Garg P, Verma A, Malik V, Maccune ER, Vasudeva A.** Dentinal Tubule Disinfection with Propolis & Two Extracts of Azadirachta indica Against Candida albicans Biofilm Formed on Tooth Substrate.
Open Dent J 2015;9:369-74.

80. **Kamath U, Sheth H, Ramesh S, Singla K.**
Comparison of the antibacterial efficacy of tea tree oil with 3% sodium hypochlorite and 2% Chlorhexidine against E. faecalis: An in vitro
study.
J Contemp dentistry 2013;3(3):117-20.

81. **Kandaswamy D, Venkateshbabu N, Gogulnath D, Kindo AJ.** Dentinal tubule disinfection with 2% chlorhexidine gel, propolis, morinda citrifolia juice, 2% povidone iodine, and calcium hydroxide. Int Endod J 2010;43(5):419-23.

82. **Khandelwal A, Ajitha P.**
Assessment of knowledge, attitude, and practice toward use of herbal medicine in endodontics among dentists in Chennai.
Drug Invention Today 2018;10:3437-42.

83. **Kulkarni G, Podar R, Singh S et al .**
Comparative evaluation of dissolution of a new resin-coated Gutta- percha, by three naturally available solvents.
Endodontology 2016;28:143-7.

84. **Le Van C, Thi Thu HP, Sangvanich P, Chuenchompoonut V, Thunyakitpisal P.**
Acemannan induces rapid early osseous defect healing after apical surgery: A 12-month follow-up of a randomized controlled trial.
J Dent Sci 2020;15(3):302-9.

85. **Mahal NK, Singh N, Thomas AM, Kakkar N.**
Effect of three different storage media on survival of periodontal ligament cells using collagenase-dispase assay.
Int Endod J 2013;46(4):365-70.

86. **Mahdi A, AL-Huwaizi HF, Abbas IS.**
A comparative evaluation of antimicrobial activity of the ethanolic extract of Cinnamomum zeylanicum and NaOCl against oral pathogens and against swabs taken from nonvital teeth - An in vitro study.
Int J Chemtech Res 2017;10 :39-47.

87. **Makarska-Białokoz M.**
History and significance of phytotherapy in the human history.
Arch Phys Glob Res 2020; 24 (2): 17-22.

88. **Mandroli PS, Prabhakar AR, Bhat K, Krishnamurthy S, Bogar C.** An in vitro evaluation of cytotoxicity of curcumin against human periodontal ligament fibroblasts.
Ayu 2019;40(3):192-5.

89. **Manjunatha M, Kini A.**
Botanicals in endodontics: A review.
J Adv Cli Res Insights 2016;3:173-6.

90. **Marcoux E.**
Antibacterial properties towards Enterococcus faecalis and safety of four natural compounds and nisin: an in vitro study [Thesis]. Laval : Laval University, 2019.

91. **Margono A, Angellina AN, Suprastiwi E.**
The effect of grape seed extraction irrigation solution towards cleanliness the smear layer on apical third of the root canal wall.
J Int Dent Med Res 2017;10(2):244-7.

92. **Martin MP, Pileggi R.**
A quantitative analysis of Propolis: a promising new storage media following avulsion.
Dent Traumatol 2004;20:85-9.

93. **Martos J, Bassotto AP, González-Rodríguez MP, Ferrer-Luque CM.** Dissolving efficacy of eucalyptus and orange oil, xylol and chloroform solvents on different root canal sealers.
Int Endod J 2011;44(11):1024-8.

94. **Matoug-Elwerfelli M, Nazzal H, Duggal M, El-Gendy R.** What the future holds for regenerative endodontics: novel antimicrobials and regenerative strategies.
Eur Cell Mater 2021;41:811-33.

95. **Mittal A, Tejaswi S, Mruthunjaya K, Shetty S, Ambikathanaya UK.** Comparison of antibacterial activity of calcium hydroxide, azadirachta indica (Neem), ocimum tenuiflorum

(Tulsi) and punica granatum (Pomegranate) gels as intracanal medicaments against Enterococcus
faecalis: An in-vitro study.
Pharmacog J 2021;13: 988-94.

96. Mittal R, Rathee G, Tandan M.
Evaluation of Antimicrobial Efficacy of Commercially Available Herbal Products as Irrigants and Medicaments in Primary Endodontics
Infections: In Vivo Study.
World J Dent 2021;11:488-93.

97. Moezizadeh M, Javand F. Tabatabaei F.
Effects of extracts of Salvadora persica on proliferation and viability of human dental pulp stem cells.
J Conserv Dent 2015;18(4):315-20.

98. Mohammad SG, Raheel SA, Baroudi K.
Histological Evaluation of Allium sativum Oil as a New Medicament for Pulp Treatment of Permanent Teeth.
J Contemp Dent Pract 2015;16(2):85-90.

99. Mohan S, Gurtu A, Singhal A, Vinayak V.
Naturopathy and endodontics-A synergistic approach.
J Dent Sci Oral Rehabil 2012;1:27-9.

100. Mookhtiar H, Hegde V, Shanmugasundaram S, Chopra MA, Kauser MN, Khan A.
Herbal Irrigants: A literataure Review Herbal Irrigants; A new Era in Endodontics: Literature Review.
Int J Dent Med Sci Res 2019;3:15-22.

101. Mukunda DA.
Efficacy of Psidium guajava leaf extract on Streptococcus mutans and Enterococcus faecalis-an in vitro study.
J Med Sci Clin Res 2019;7 :752-8.

102. Murray PE, Farber RM, Namerow KN, Kuttler S, Garcia-Godoy F.
Evaluation of Morinda citrifolia as an endodontic irrigant.
J Endod 2008;34(1):66-70.

103. Neelakantan P, Cheng CQ, Ravichandran V et al. Photoactivation of curcumin and sodium hypochlorite to enhance antibiofilm efficacy in root canal dentin.
Photodiagnosis Photodyn Ther 2015;12(1):108-14.

104. Nosrat A, Bolhari B, Sharifian MR, Aligholi M, Mortazavi MS. The effect of Carvacrol on Enterococcus faecalis as a final irrigant. Iran Endod J 2009;4(3):96-100.

105. Omar OM, Khattab NM, Khater DS.
Nigella sativa oil as a pulp medicament for pulpotomized teeth: a histopathological evaluation.
J Clin Pediatr Dent 2012;36(4):335-41.

106. **Ozan F, Polat ZA, Er K, Ozan U, Değer O.**
Effect of propolis on survival of periodontal ligament cells: new storage media for avulsed teeth.
J Endod 2007;33(5):570-3.

107. **Pagliarin CM, Londero L, Felippe MC, Felippe WT, Danesi CC, Barletta FB.**
Tissue characterization following revascularization of immature dog teeth using different disinfection pastes.
Braz Oral Res. 2016;30(1):1-10.

108. **Pandey S, Shekhar R, Paul R, Hans M, Garg A.**
A comparative evaluation and effectiveness of different antimicrobial herbal extracts as endodontic irrigants against Enterococcus faecalis and Candida albicans-An in-vitro study.
University J Dent Sci. 2018;4:75-8.

109. **Parolia A, Kundabala M, Rao NN et al.**
A comparative histological analysis of human pulp following direct pulp capping with Propolis, mineral trioxide aggregate and Dycal. Aust Dent J 2010;55(1):59-64.

110. **Pathak SD, Bansode PV, Wavdhane MB, Khedgikar SB, Pandey A.**
Phytotherapeutics and Endodontics-A Review.
J Med Dent Sci Res 2017;4:29-31.

111. **Pereira JV, Bergamo DC, Pereira JO, França Sde C, Pietro RC, Silva- Sousa YT.**
Antimicrobial activity of Arctium lappa constituents against microorganisms commonly found in endodontic infections. Braz Dent J 2005;16(3):192-6.

112. **Pithon MM, Lacerda-Santos R, Oliveira GC, et al.**
Effect of different combinations of papain-based gels on dissolving pulp tissue.
Biosci J 2017;33 :1099-105.

113. **Prabhakar J, Senthilkumar M, Priya MS, Mahalakshmi K, Sehgal PK, Sukumaran VG.**
Evaluation of antimicrobial efficacy of herbal alternatives (Triphala and green tea polyphenols), MTAD, and 5% sodium hypochlorite
against Enterococcus faecalis biofilm formed on tooth substrate: an in vitro study.
J Endod 2010;36(1):83-6.

114. **Priyangha V, Kumar S, Ramesh S.**
Antibacterial Efficacy of Psidium Guajava Leaf Extract on E. feacalis-In Vitro Study.
Ann Med Health Sci Res 2021;11 :81-6.

115. **Purohit RN, Bhatt M, Purohit K, Acharya J, Kumar R, Garg R.** Clinical and Radiological Evaluation of Turmeric Powder as a Pulpotomy Medicament in Primary Teeth: An in vivo Study.
Int J Clin Pediatr Dent 2017;10(1):37-40.

116. **Qi J, Gong M, Zhang R et al.**
Evaluation of the antibacterial effect of tea tree oil on Enterococcus faecalis and biofilm in vitro.
J Ethnopharmacol 2021;281:1-10.

117. **Rani A, Thakur S, Gupta S, Gauniyal P, Bhandari M, Gupta H.**
Comparative Evaluation Of Antimicrobial Activity Of Different Herbal Extracts And 2% Chlorhexidine Gluconate Against E. Faecalis & C. Albicans: An In Vitro Study.
Indian J Dent Sci 2015;7:20-3.

118. **Reddy JM, Sandhya R.**
Antimicrobial efficacy of neem, calcium hydroxide and combination of both as an intracanal medicament against e. faecalis-an in vitro study. plant cell biotechnology and molecular biology.
Plant Cell Biotechnol Mol Biol 2020;21(25-26): 88-95.

119. **Rehman K, Khan FR, Aman N.**
Comparison of orange oil and chloroform as gutta- percha solvents in endodontic retreatment.
J Contemp Dent Pract 2013;14(3):478-82.

120. **Reiznautt CM, Ribeiro JS, Kreps E et al.**
Development and properties of endodontic resin sealers with natural oils.
J Dent 2021;104:1-7.

121. **Sabir A, Tabbu CR, Agustiono P, Sosroseno W.**
Histological analysis of rat dental pulp tissue capped with propolis.
J Oral Sci 2005;47(3):135-8.

122. **Saghiri MA, García-Godoy F, Asgar K, Lotfi M.**
The effect of Morinda Citrifolia juice as an endodontic irrigant on smear layer and microhardness of root canal dentin.
Oral Sci Int 2013;10(2):53-7.

123. **Sahebi S, Khosravifar N, Sedighshamsi M, Motamedifar M.** Comparison of the antibacterial effect of sodium hypochlorite and aloe vera solutions as root canal irrigants in human extracted teeth contaminated with enterococcus faecalis.
J Dent 2014; 15(1):39-43.

124. **Sarrami N, Pemberton MN, Thornhill MH, Theaker ED.**
Adverse reactions associated with the use of eugenol in dentistry.
Br Dent J 2002; 193(5):257-9.

125. **Seal M, Rishi R, Satish G, Divya KT, Talukdar P, Maniyar R.**
Herbal panacea: The need for today in dentistry. J Int Soc Prev Community Dent 2016;6(2):105-9.

126. **Sebatni MA, Kumar AA.**
Smear layer removal efficacy of herbal extracts used as endodontic irrigants: An: in vitro: study.
Endodontology 2017;29(1):35-8.

127. **Setty JV, Srinivasan I, Sathiesh RT, Kale M, Shetty VV, Venkatesh S.** In vitro evaluation of antimicrobial effect of Myristica fragrans on common endodontic pathogens.
J Indian Soc Pedod Prev Dent 2020;38(2):145-51.

128. **Shabbir J, Najmi N, Zehra T ,Ali S, Khurshid Z, Zafar MS, Palma PJ.**
Intracanal drugs.
Biomaterials in Endodontics 2022: 5-81.

129. **Shabbir J, Qazi F, Farooqui W, Ahmed S, Zehra T, Khurshid Z.**
Effect of Chinese Propolis as an Intracanal Medicament on Post-...
Operative Endodontic Pain: A Double-Blind Randomized Controlled Trial.
Int J Environ Res Public Health 2020;17(2):1-10.

130. **Siddique R, Ranjan M, Jose J, Srivastav A, Rajakeerthi R, Kamath A.** Clinical
Quantitative Antibacterial Potency of Garlic-Lemon Against Sodium Hypochlorite in Infected
Root Canals: A Double-blinded, Randomized, Controlled Clinical Trial.
J Int Soc Prev Community Dent 2020;10(6):771-8.

131. **Silva FB, Almeida JM, Sousa SM.**
Natural medicaments in endodontics -- a comparative study of the anti-inflammatory action.
Braz Oral Res 2004; 18(2):174-9.

132. **Singh S, Das D.**
Passion fruit: a fetched passion for dentists.
Int J Pharm Sci Res 2013; 4(2):754-7.

133. **Sinha DJ, Sinha AA.**
Natural medicines in dentistry.
Ayu 2014;35(2):113-8.

134. **Sinha DJ, Vasudeva A, Jaiswal N, Garg P, Tyagi SP, Singh J.** Antibacterial
efficacy of Melaleuca alternifolia (Tea tree oil), Curcuma longa (Turmeric), 2%
chlorhexidine, and 5% sodium hypochlorite against Enterococcus faecalis: An in vitro study.
Saudi Endod J 2015;5:182-6.

135. **Sivakumar A, Ravi V, Prasad AS, Sivakumar JS.** Herbendodontics-Phytotherapy in
endodontics: A review. Biomed Pharm J 2018;11:1073-82.

136. **Soligo LT, Lodi E, Farina AP, Souza MA, Vidal C, Cecchin D.** Antibacterial
Efficacy of Synthetic and Natural-Derived Novel Endodontic Irrigant Solutions.
Braz Den J 2018;29(5):459-64.

137. **Songsiripradubboon S, Banlunara W, Sangvanich P, Trairatvorakul C,
Thunyakitpisal P.** Clinical, radiographic, and histologic analysis of the effects of acemannan
used in direct pulp capping of human primary teeth: short-term outcomes. Odontology
2016;104(3):329-37.

138. **Songsiripradubboon S, Kladkaew S, Trairatvorakul C et al.** Stimulation of Dentin
Regeneration by Using Acemannan in Teeth with Lipopolysaccharide-induced Pulp
Inflammation.
J Endod 2017;43(7):1097-103.

139. **Souza BD, Alves AM, Santos LG, Simões CM, Felippe WT, Felippe MC.**
Fibroblast Viability after Storage at 20 °C in Milk, Hank's Balanced Salt Solution and
Coconut Water.
Braz Dent J 2016;27(4):404-7.

140. **Sowjanyaa J, Thomas T, Chandana CS.**
Comparative evaluation of the efficacy of smear layer removal by ethylenediaminetetraacetic acid, Triphala, and German chamomile as irrigants - A scanning electron microscopy study. J Adv Pharm Educ Res 2017;7(3) :267-71.

141. **Subramaniam T, Subramaniam A, Chowdhery A, Das S, Gill M.**
Versatility of aloe vera in dentistry-a review.
J Dent Med Sci 2014; 13:98-102.

142. **Tafazoli Moghadam E, Yazdanian M, Alam M et al.**
Current natural bioactive materials in bone and tooth regeneration in dentistry: a comprehensiveoverview.
J Materials Res Technol 2021;13:2078-114.

143. **Tewari RK, Kapoor B, Mishra SK, Kumar A.**
Role of herbs in endodontics.
J Oral Res Rev 2016;8(2):95-9.

144. **Tonea A, Badea M, Oana L, Sava S, Vodnar D.**
Antibacterial and antifungal activity of endodontic intracanal medications.
Clujul Med 2017;90(3):344-7.

145. **Tyagi SP, Sinha DJ, Garg P, Singh UP, Mishra CC, Nagpal R.** Comparison of antimicrobial efficacy of propolis, Morinda citrifolia, Azadirachta indica (Neem) and 5% sodium hypochlorite on Candida albicans biofilm formed on tooth substrate: An in-vitro study.
J Conserv Dent 2013;16(6):532-5.

146. **Venkataram V, Gokhale ST, Kenchappa M, Nagarajappa R.**
Effectiveness of chamomile (Matricaria recutita L.), MTAD and sodium hypochlorite irrigants on smear layer.
Eur Arch Paediatr Dent 2013;14:247-52.

147. **Venkateshbabu N, Anand S, Abarajithan M, Sheriff SO, Jacob PS, Sonia N.**
Natural Therapeutic Options in Endodontics - A Review.
Open Dent J 2016;10:214-26.

148. **Vishwanath V, Rao HM.**
Gutta-percha in endodontics - A comprehensive review of material science.
J Conserv Dent 2019; 22(3):216-22.

149. **Vu NB, Chuenchompoonut V, Jansisyanont P, Sangvanich P, Pham TH, Thunyakitpisal P.**
Acemannan-induced tooth socket healing: A 12-month randomized controlled trial.
J Dent Sci 2021; 16(2):643-53.

150. **Vu TT, Nguyen MT, Sangvanich P, Nguyen QN, Thunyakitpisal P.**
Acemannan Used as an Implantable Biomaterial for Vital Pulp Therapy of Immature Permanent Teeth Induced Continued Root Formation.
Pharmaceutics 2020;12(7):1-15

151. **Widjiastuti I, Saraswati W, Rahma A.**
The Role of Propolis in Pulp Pain by Inhibiting Cyclooxygenase-2 Expression.
Conserv Dent J 2021; 11(1):11-8.

152. **Więckiewicz W, Miernik M, Więckiewicz M, Morawiec T.**
Does Propolis Help to Maintain Oral Health?
Evid Based Complement Alternat Med 2013;2013:1-8.

153. **Winarni Y, Haslinda R, Aspalilah A.**
Miswak: The underutilised device and future challenges.
J Dent Oral Hyg 2019;11(2):6-11.

154. **Xue W, Yu J, Chen W.**
Plants and Their Bioactive Constituents in Mesenchymal Stem Cell- Based Periodontal
Regeneration: A Novel Prospective.
Biomed Res Int 2018;2018:173-6.

155. **Yuanita T, Zubaidah N, Kunarti S.**
Expression of Osteoprotegrin and Osteoclast Level in Chronic Apical Periodontitis Induced
with East Java Propolis Extract.
Iran Endod J 2018;13(1):42-6.

156. **Zohery AA, Meshri SM, Madi MI, Abd El Rehim SS, Nour ZM.** Egyptian propolis
compared to nanohydroxyapatite graft in the treatment of Class II furcation defects in dogs.
J Periodontol 2018; 89:1340-50.

157. **Zulhendri F, Felitti R, Fearnley J, Ravalia M.**
The use of propolis in dentistry, oral health, and medicine: A review.
J Oral Biosci 2021;63(1):23-34.

Internet references

158. **Grandma's tips.**
Natural remedies, tips and recipes [Online].
[Accessed 28/04/2023], available from the URL: https://astucesdegrandmere.net/mal-de-dents-
remedes-calmer- pain

159. **Creapharma.**
Thyme flowers [Online].
[Accessed 28/04/2023], available from the URL:
https://www.creapharma.ch/thym.htm

160. **Devaux G.**
7 scientifically proven benefits of peppermint [Online]. [Accessed on 28/04/2023], available
from the URL: https://www.auparadisduthe.com/blog/bienfaits-menthe-poivree/

161. **Doctissimo.**
Tulsi (Ocimum tenuiflorum or Ocinum sanctum) [Online]. [Accessed on 28/04/2023],
available from the URL: https://www.doctissimo.fr/medecines-douces/medecine-
ayurvedique/principales-plantes-ayurvediques/tulsi-ocimum- tenuiflorum

162. **Ecosostenibile**.

Bixa orellana: Systematics, Etymology, Habitat, Cultivation [Online]. [Accessed on 28/04/2023], available from the URL: https://antropocene.it/en/2023/01/10/bixa-orellana-2/

163. **Emci**.

Essential oil of Tagetes (Tagetes minuta) [Online]. [Accessed on 28/04/2023], available from URL: https://www.huileessentielle-bio.com/huile-essentielle-tagete- tagetes-minuta/

154. **Freepik**

Citron [Online].

[Accessed 28/04/2023], available from the URL:

https://fr.freepik.com/photos/citron-jaune

155. **National Natural Heritage Inventory (INPN)**.

Casearia sylvestris Sw [Online].

[Accessed 28/04/2023], available from the URL:

https://inpn.mnhn.fr/espece/cd_nom/629277

156. **Gardening**.

German chamomile flowers [Online].

[Accessed 28/04/2023], available from the URL:

https://jardinage.lemonde.fr/dossier-1785-matricaire-matricaria recutita.html

157. **Gardening**.

Neem fruits and leaves [Online].

[Accessed 28/04/2023], available from the URL: https://jardinage.lemonde.fr/dossier-3579-neem margousier-tres- ancien-remede-ayurvedique.html

168. **Lecourrier**.

Myrtle [Online].

[Accessed 28/04/2023], available from the URL:

https://lecourrier.vn/le-myrte/473356.html

169. **Lefaso**.

Acacia Nilotica [Online].

[Accessed on 28/04/2023], available from the URL: https://lefaso.net/spip.php?article48128

170. **Logees**.

Cinnamon leaves [Online].

[Accessed 28/04/2023], available from the URL:

https://www.logees.com/cinnamon-cinnamomum zeylanicum.html

171. **Marqueverte**.

Aloe vera leaves [Online].

[Accessed 28/04/2023], available from the URL: https://www.marqueverte.com/blog/aloe-vera-une-plante-medicinale- aux-multiples vertus-en-cosmetique-n529

172. **Nutrilife shop**.

La papaïne: Une acide précieuse " fructueuse " [On line]. [Accessed on 28/04/2023], available from the URL: https://blog.nutrilifeshop.com/la-papaine/

173. **Olfastory**.

Parfum Noix de muscade, Nutmeg in perfumery [Online]. [Accessed on 28/04/2023], available from the URL: https://www.olfastory.com/matiere/noix-de-muscade

174. **Passportante**.

Curcuma : frais ou moulu, toutes les vertus de cet épice [On line]. [Accessed 28/04/2023], available from the URL: https://www.passeportsante.net/fr/Nutrition/EncyclopedieAliments/Fiche.aspx?doc=curcuma_nu

175. **Pinterest**.

Passion fruit [Online].

[Accessed 28/04/2023], available from the URL:

https://www.pinterest.fr/pin/59039445103991204/4

176. **Plants and Health**.

Black cumin against covid-19 [Online].

[Accessed on 28/04/2023], available from the URL: https://www.plantes-et-sante.fr/articles/phytotherapie/3965-covid-19- la-nigelle-a-raison-de-faire-parler-delle

177. **Proteins**.

administrator. Grape seed extract [Online].

[Accessed on 28/04/2023], available from the URL: https://proteines-vegetales.fr/extrait-de-pepins-de-raisin/

178. **Health Science**.

Camellia sinensis : Analysis of its health properties and virtues [Online].

[Accessed 28/04/2023], available from the URL:

https://www.santescience.fr/camellia-sinensis/

179. **All articles**.

Noni juice guide map [Online].

[Accessed on 28/04/2023], available from the URL: https://www.jus- de-noni.net/site-plan/

180. **Wikipedia**.

Carvacrol [Online].

[Accessed 28/04/2023], available from the URL:

https://fr.wikipedia.org/w/index.php?title=Carvacrol&oldid=200010 127

181. **Wikipedia**.

Copaifera [Online].

[Accessed 28/04/2023], available from the URL:

https://fr.wikipedia.org/w/index.php?title=Copaifera&oldid=203052 960

182. **Wikipedia**.

Cumin [Internet]. 2022 [cited 6 May 2023]. Available from:

https://fr.wikipedia.org/w/index.php?title=Cumin&oldid=196526811

183. **Wikipedia**.

Gum ferrule [On line].

[Accessed 28/04/2023], available from the URL:

https://fr.wikipedia.org/w/index.php?title=F%C3%A9rule_gommeus e&oldid=184387320

184. **Wikipedia**.

Great burdock [Online].

[Accessed 28/04/2023], available from the URL:

https://fr.wikipedia.org/w/index.php?title=Grande_bardane&oldid=2 00753527

185. **Wikipedia**.

Castor oil [Online].

[Accessed 28/04/2023], available from the URL:
https://fr.wikipedia.org/w/index.php?title=Huile_de_ricin&oldid=203 789920

186. **Wikipedia**.

Propolis [Online].

[Accessed on 28/04/2023], available from the URL:
https://fr.wikipedia.org/w/index.php?title=Propolis&oldid=203786904

187. **Wikipedia**.

Psidium guajava [Online].

[Accessed on 28/04/2023], available from the URL:
https://en.wikipedia.org/w/index.php?title=Psidium_guajava&oldid= 1145378948

188. **Wikipedia**.

Set [Online].

[Accessed 28/04/2023], available from the URL:

https://fr.wikipedia.org/w/index.php?title=R%C3%A9glisse&oldid=2 02790190

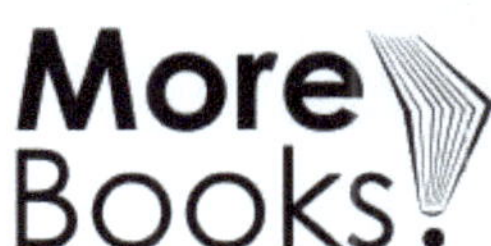

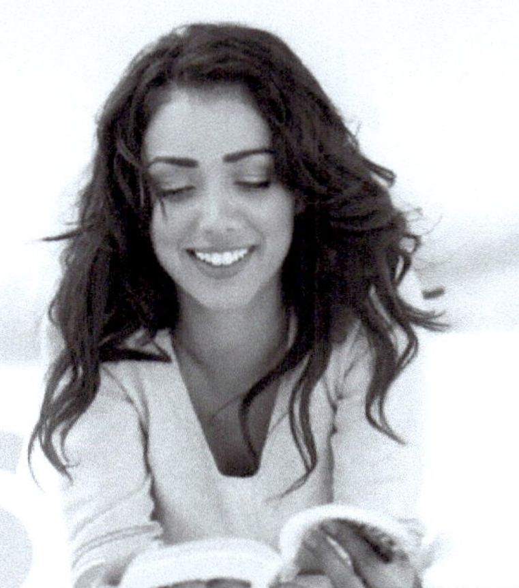

I want morebooks!

Buy your books fast and straightforward online - at one of world's fastest growing online book stores! Environmentally sound due to Print-on-Demand technologies.

Buy your books online at
www.morebooks.shop

Kaufen Sie Ihre Bücher schnell und unkompliziert online – auf einer der am schnellsten wachsenden Buchhandelsplattformen weltweit! Dank Print-On-Demand umwelt- und ressourcenschonend produziert.

Bücher schneller online kaufen
www.morebooks.shop

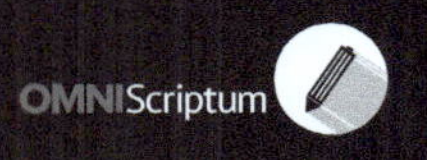

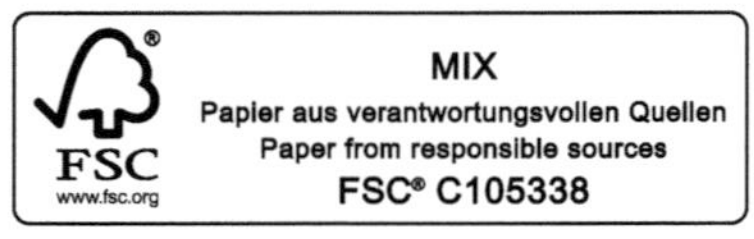